D1607195

Little, Brown's Paperback Book Series

Basic Medical Sciences

Borysenko et al.	Functional Histology
Boyd & Hoerl	Basic Medical Microbiology
Colton	Statistics in Medicine
Daube et al.	Medical Neurosciences
Friedman	Biochemistry
Kent	General Pathology: A Programmed Text
Levine	Pharmacology
Miller	Peery and Miller's Pathology
Reich	Hematology (Physiopathology series)
Richardson	Basic Circulatory Physiology
Roland et al.	Atlas of Cell Biology
Selkurt	Physiology
Sidman & Sidman	Neuroanatomy: A Programmed Text
Siegel, Albers, et al.	Basic Neurochemistry
Snell	Clinical Anatomy for Medical Students
Snell	Clinical Embryology for Medical Students
Streilein & Hughes	Immunology: A Programmed Text
Valtin	Renal Dysfunction (Physiopathology series)
Valtin	Renal Function
Watson	Basic Human Neuroanatomy

Clinical Medical Sciences

Clark & MacMahon	Preventive Medicine
Eckert	Emergency-Room Care
Grabb & Smith	Plastic Surgery
Green	Gynecology
Gregory & Smeltzer	Psychiatry
Judge & Zuidema	Methods of Clinical Examination
Nardi & Zuidema	Surgery
Niswander	Obstetrics
Thompson	Primer of Clinical Radiology
Wilkins & Levinsky	Medicine
Ziai	Pediatrics

Manuals and Handbooks

Alpert & Francis	Manual of Coronary Care
Arndt	Manual of Dermatologic Therapeutics
Berk et al.	Handbook of Critical Care
Bochner et al.	Handbook of Clinical Pharmacology
Children's Hospital Medical Center, Boston	Manual of Pediatric Therapeutics
Condon & Nyhus	Manual of Surgical Therapeutics
Friedman	Problem-Oriented Medical Diagnosis
Gantz & Gleckman	Manual of Clinical Problems in Infectious Diseases: With Annotated Key References
Gardner & Provine	Manual of Acute Bacterial Infections
Iversen & Clawson	Manual of Orthopaedic Therapeutics
Klippel & Anderson	Manual of Emergency and Outpatient Techniques
Leaverton	A Review of Biostatistics: A Program for Self-Instruction
Massachusetts General Hospital	Clinical Anesthesia Procedures
Papper	Manual of Medical Care of the Surgical Patient
Roberts	Manual of Clinical Problems in Pediatrics: With Annotated Key References
Samuels	Manual of Neurologic Therapeutics
Shader	Manual of Psychiatric Therapeutics
Snow	Manual of Anesthesia
Spivak & Barnes	Manual of Clinical Problems in Internal Medicine: Annotated with Key References
Wallach	Interpretation of Diagnostic Tests
Washington University Department of Medicine	Manual of Medical Therapeutics
Zimmerman	Techniques of Patient Care

Manual of Emergency
and Outpatient Techniques

EDITED BY

Allen P. Klippel, M.D.
Associate Professor of Surgery,
Creighton University School of Medicine;
Director, Emergency Department,
Creighton Memorial–Saint Joseph's Hospital, Omaha, Nebraska;
formerly Assistant Professor of Surgery,
Washington University School of Medicine,
St. Louis, Missouri

Charles B. Anderson, M.D.
Associate Professor of Surgery,
Washington University School of Medicine;
Associate Surgeon,
Barnes Hospital, St. Louis, Missouri

Manual of Emergency and Outpatient Techniques

Washington University Department of Surgery

LITTLE, BROWN AND COMPANY   BOSTON

Figure, page 165 (bottom): modified from F. Plum and J. B. Posner, *The Diagnosis of Stupor and Coma.* Copyright © 1972 by F. A. Davis Co., Philadelphia.

Figures, pages 326–329, 331: modified from J. R. Willson, *Atlas of Obstetric Technic,* 2nd ed. St. Louis: The C. V. Mosby Company, 1969. Original artwork in *Atlas* by Daisy Stilwell.

This book is dedicated to our wives

Mary and Marilynn

Preface

This manual is designed to familiarize medical students, house officers, physicians, and other medical personnel who work in emergency areas with many of the techniques required for emergency and outpatient surgical management. Primarily, basic procedures are covered, but since some more sophisticated techniques are presented, it must not be construed that all the procedures can be performed by less than trained surgeons. However, surgical technicians, medical students, and house officers should be familiar with the operations and procedures at which they are expected to assist.

Surgical diagnosis and treatment must always be kept paramount, but there are important technical aspects to surgery and emergency medicine that cannot be ignored. Carrying out a procedure improperly is often worse than not attempting it at all. The patient who suffers a pneumothorax as a result of a misplaced central venous catheter now has an additional obstacle to survival. It is the expectation of the contributors to this manual that they may impart some of the skills they have learned during the complex technical management of today's surgical patient, in the hope that certain pitfalls may be avoided.

This manual has been prepared by members of the Washington University School of Medicine, St. Louis, Missouri. We are especially grateful for the advice and guidance of Dr. Walter F. Ballinger, Professor of Surgery and formerly Chairman of the Department of Surgery. The editors appreciate the assistance and direction provided by Mr. Fred Belliveau and his staff at Little, Brown and Company, and recognize the untiring efforts of Ms. Bernice Flynn and Ms. Lynell Conley, who quietly and uncomplainingly typed and retyped the manuscript.

A. P. K.
C. B. A.

Contents

Manual of Emergency
and Outpatient Techniques

Notice

The indications and dosages of all drugs in this book have been recommended in the medical literature and conform to practices of the general medical community at Washington University. The medications described do not necessarily have specific approval by the Food and Drug Administration for use in the diseases and dosages for which they are recommended. The package insert for each drug should be consulted for use and dosage as approved by the FDA. Because standards for usage change, it is advisable to keep abreast of revised recommendations, particularly those concerning new drugs.

1

Patient Handling

Allen P. Klippel

It is appropriate to begin a book on the technical aspects of outpatient surgery with a discussion of some of the most important techniques used on our patients. For too long it has been considered that professional medical management begins at the entrance to the emergency department. Only recently has it become obvious that inept initial handling of the patient on the scene of the accident or illness can frustrate the later application of the best skills of the medical profession. This chapter therefore is designed not only to help the in-house personnel in patient handling but also to encourage them to involve themselves in what transpires before the patient arrives, including the teaching of paramedical personnel. Training in the fundamentals of first aid and rescue should be mandatory for all medical students, nurses, and other medical personnel. The emergency manual, prepared by the American Academy of Orthopedic Surgeons, is an excellent text for such training. Hospital personnel need to be familiar with the techniques used in patient handling on the accident scene to make the patient comfortable and avoid increased injury, since these techniques are also needed in the hospital environment for the same reasons. If hospital personnel understand the work of rescue personnel, they will learn *not* to remove splints or backboards before the indicated examinations and roentgenograms have been made.

Every emergency department should stock the same equipment that is used by the local ambulance or rescue services, so that equipment can be immediately exchanged and there is no need for the service to wait for its return. This concept was promulgated by Letterman in 1863, during the Civil War, but to date has had little use despite its obvious merit. The essential equipment list for ambulances drawn up by the American College of Surgeons is an excellent starting point. Many physicians and ambulance personnel will add other items of equipment they find useful in handling their patients.

Initial Procedures
AIRWAY CONTROL
Establishment and maintenance of an adequate airway is the most important step in handling any patient who is not breathing normally.

WOUNDS AND HEMORRHAGE

Every open wound should be covered by a sterile dry gauze dressing. Larger wounds may be covered with multilayered gauze dressings. These dressings are held in place with triangular bandages or conforming gauze roller bandage. This direct pressure will control almost all types of hemorrhage except that from a severed major artery.

If a dressing becomes soaked with blood, more pads should be applied and wrapped snugly with a conforming gauze roller bandage or air splint. An air splint not only will splint an extremity but also is an excellent method of controlling hemorrhage. The initial bandage must not be removed.

A tourniquet should be used only as a last resort when bleeding can be stopped in *no* other way. Loss of an extremity must be anticipated if a tourniquet is applied. The tourniquet should be wide enough so that it applies pressure as a wide band and does not damage underlying nerves and vessels. A stick or pencil is inserted in the tourniquet and twisted until the wound is absolutely dry. *Do not loosen the tourniquet until definitive wound management is available.*

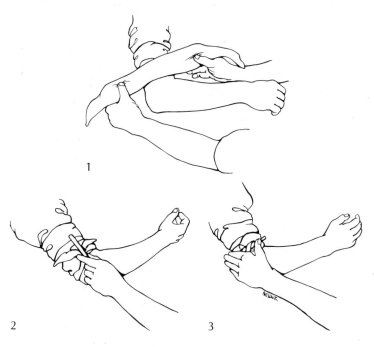

1

2

3

EMERGENCY SPLINTING

Any suspected fracture site must be splinted as soon as possible and before transport to the hospital, even if the hospital is close by. The general principle that must be followed is that the joints proximal and distal to the fracture site must be included in the splinting. Hospital personnel are all too familiar with the delays that some fracture patients must undergo in the x-ray department or waiting for a cast to be applied, especially when more seriously ill or injured patients arrive. The neurologic and vascular state of the extremity must be evaluated before and after a splint has been applied, to rule out any deleterious effects of the splint.

Shoulder Girdle and Upper Arm

A fractured clavicle is splinted by pulling back the shoulders and holding the position with two triangular bandages tied together or a 4-inch conforming gauze roll applied to the patient in a figure-eight technique. The patient will be more comfortable if the anterior axillary fold is padded with a multilayered gauze pad on each side.

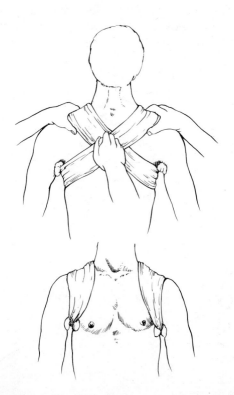

Fractures of the shoulder area are best managed by placing the arm in a sling and tying a second triangular bandage around the body.

Two long, well-padded boards may be used for fractures of the humerus when the elbow cannot be flexed. These are applied while gentle traction is exerted on the hand.

Forearm

Padded board splints and a sling are used for fractures of the forearm. A long air splint can be used for fractures of the forearm or elbow that cannot be flexed. An air splint can be used for fractures at the distal end of the forearm or wrist, but care must be taken that the fingers do not project beyond the splint and thereby become edematous.

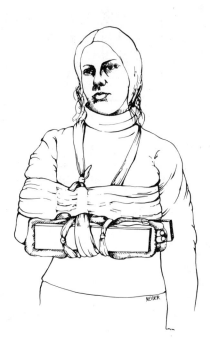

Only those air splints that open along their length should be used because they are most easily applied.

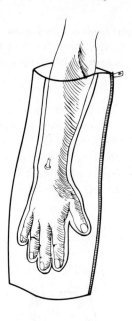

Hands

All fractures of the bones of the hand must be splinted in the anatomic position. A roller bandage is placed in the palm and the fingers fitted around it. The extremity is then placed on a padded board splint or short air splint.

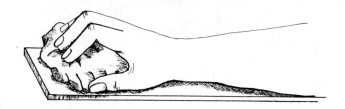

Upper Leg

HIP. Fractures of the hip or pelvis are probably best handled by tying the two legs together and carrying the patient on a long backboard or scoop litter.

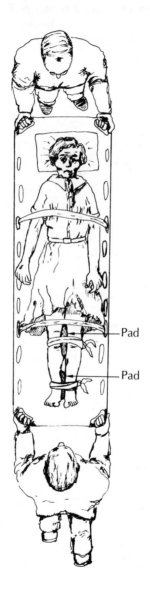

Pad

Pad

FEMUR. The half ring splint must be applied so that the padded ring impinges on the ischial tuberosity, not on the pubic bone. As one rescuer provides traction at the foot, the splint is slipped into position. The patient's shoe is left on, and traction is applied by an ankle hitch using a triangular bandage. The hitch is tightened by a spanish windless stick that is held in place with adhesive tape. Triangular bandages are used to hold the leg. The foot and ankle must be elevated.

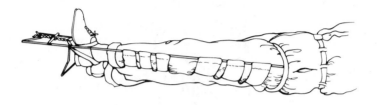

Commercial versions of the half ring splint are usually quickly applied, since Velco leg supports, foot-traction straps, and a heel rest are all attached to the splint.

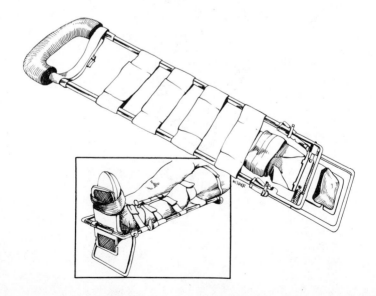

KNEE. Fractures about the knee may be handled with a half ring splint, long leg air splint, or long padded board splints.

Lower Leg

Fractures of the lower leg are splinted with long-leg air splints or long padded board splints.

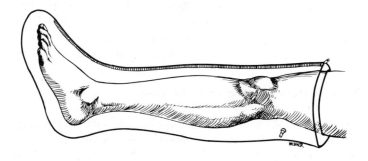

ANKLE AND FOOT. Ankle or foot fractures can be splinted by an air splint or by wrapping a blanket or pillow around the foot and ankle and tying board splints around it.

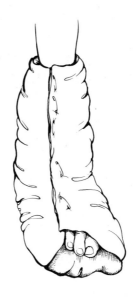

Open fractures should have a dry dressing applied to the wound and only enough traction used to allow the splint to be applied. Obviously, a fracture displaced to a great degree needs to be straightened enough to relieve the problem, especially when there is some possibility of compromising the blood supply to the distal arm or leg.

No splint or backboard of any type is to be removed to inspect the extremity or check the wound until at least preliminary roentgenograms have been made unless the splint appears to be improperly applied or hemorrhage is apparently uncontrolled.

Removal from Buildings or Excavations
LOG ROLL

The unconscious patient is rolled to one side with traction being applied to the head and neck, keeping the head aligned with the rest of the body. A long backboard is slid under the patient, and he is fastened to it. The head is sandbagged to hold the normal position.

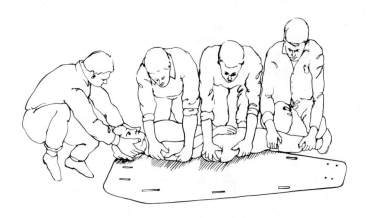

FOUR-MAN CARRY
While the patient is being carried, every effort must be made to keep the back and head in the normal anatomic position.

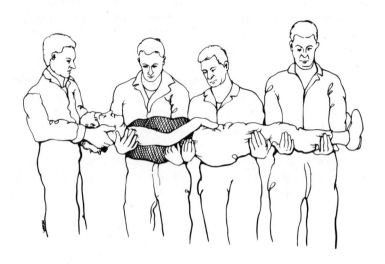

CHAIR CARRY
A patient may be strapped to a chair or to a chair litter for carrying down narrow, twisting stairs if there is no suspected vertebral column injury.

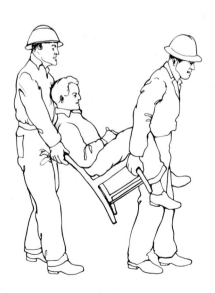

Vehicle Extrications

EXTRICATION FROM WITHIN A VEHICLE

In every wreck situation the vehicle must be stabilized and all other hazards controlled. Enough of the wreck must be cut away to allow for easy removal of the victims. There is no excuse for dragging an injured person through the windshield or window unless the vehicle is burning out of control.

One member of the rescue team must remain inside the vehicle to care for the victims by controlling the airway and stopping hemorrhage. In holding an unconscious patient's head in the anatomic position the rescuer protects both the airway and cervical spine. If the victim's head is locked in any position, no attempt should be made to correct the alignment with the body. Rather, the head should be splinted as it is by wrapping the neck with a cervical collar.

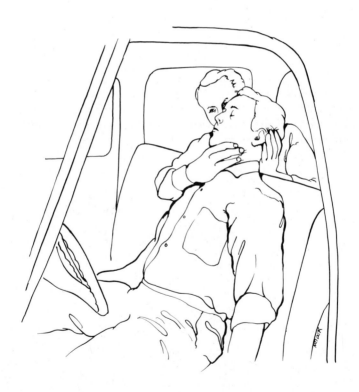

Every patient who is unconscious or who may even remotely have a spinal column injury must be fastened to a short backboard before being moved. Splinting must be done where the patient is found. The seat can be "popped" from the seat rails by a crowbar or "come-along" fastened around the seat to gain enough room to work.

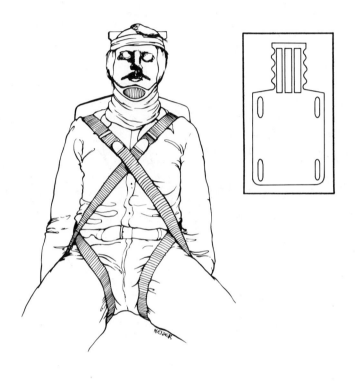

The head and neck can be stabilized by a rigid cervical collar or a chin strap. A chin strap must be avoided if there is any possibility of vomiting. The collar must be made of a material stiff enough to maintain the normal cervical curve and completely splint the neck.

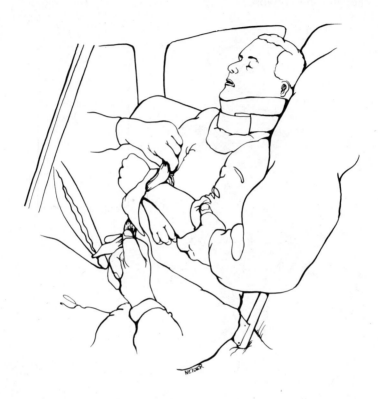

The patient is strapped to a short backboard or the upper half of the segmented board.

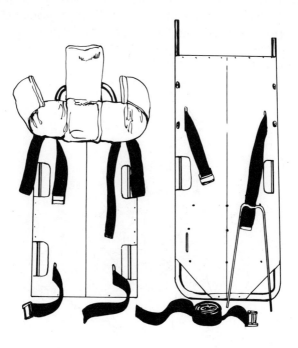

Arms and legs must be fastened together so that they cannot be entangled in the wreckage; this also provides preliminary splinting during the extrication maneuvers. When the patient has been placed on the ground, the rest of the stretcher is assembled, or he is strapped to a long board for transport. At this point it is usually necessary to readjust the various straps and to apply other needed bandages and splints.

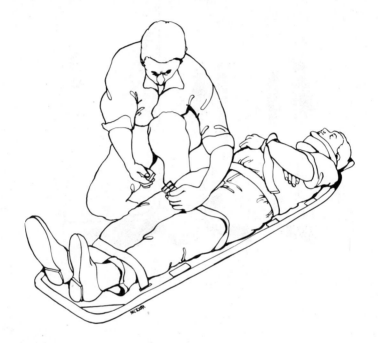

EXTRICATION FROM UNDER A VEHICLE

When a victim is trapped under a vehicle that cannot be moved, the vehicle is jacked up and blocks are inserted to maintain its position. The victim is pulled out by passing a heavy belt or rope across the upper chest and under the arms. One rescuer pulls on the head, holding the head and neck in normal anatomic alignment; the others pull on the rope that has been crisscrossed beneath the head to support it. By this traction the victim is pulled onto a long backboard.

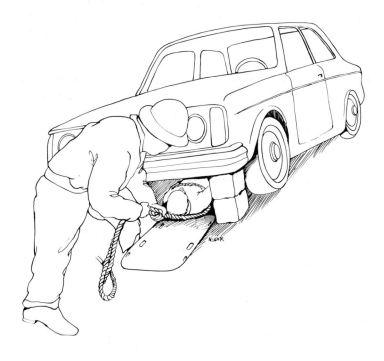

Transportation

Conscious patients are usually most comfortable when they are transported prone with a pillow under the head. However, a pillow should not be used under the head of an unconscious patient because flexing the neck tends to occlude the airway. It is essential for the rescue technician to be so situated that he can have the oxygen supply and bag mask resuscitator and the suction equipment readily available.

Oxygen can be supplied by face mask or nasal catheter. The length of the catheter is determined by measuring the distance from the tip of the nose to the earlobe and inserting the catheter only that far.

Patients with chest injuries should be transported with the damaged side down, which allows for maximal ventilation by the undamaged lung.

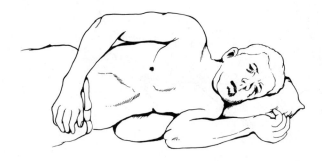

Some patients with lung or heart disease may feel better being transported in a semisitting position, and oxygen by nasal cannula or mask or by demand valve is usually helpful. A sandbag placed on the flail segment or turning the patient to lie on the sandbag will stabilize the chest by preventing paradoxical movement with consequent loss of ventilation. A flailing segment has the effect of increasing the dead air space.

Unconscious patients, especially those who have had a cerebrovascular accident, are best transported on their side in the "coma" position. In this position, vomitus runs out easily, reducing the risk of aspiration. This position is *not* recommended for patients with possible vertebral column injuries, who should be properly strapped to a long backboard.

SHOCK

If the patient is on a long backboard, the foot end may be elevated 4 to 6 inches to combat shock. However, if the patient is obese, elevating the foot end of the backboard is not recommended, since pressure on the diaphragm by the abdominal contents may limit respiratory exchange.

Three-compartment airpants are now available to manage shock resulting from profound blood loss. The pants are wrapped around the lower extremities and lower abdomen and inflated to 40 mm Hg with a foot pump. This technique will often raise the systolic pressure 40 to 60 mm Hg; it has been suggested that application of the suit is equal to the infusion of three units of blood. Care must be taken in the application of the abdominal part, to prevent compression of the upper abdomen or lower chest, which would limit respiratory excursion.

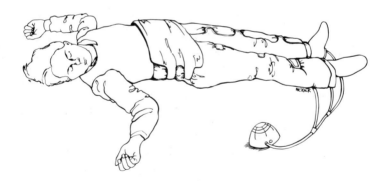

VENTILATION

It is essential that the airway be kept clear of vomitus or other materials. A good suction device should be available, including a battery-powered unit, so that it can be taken out of the ambulance and to the patient if needed.

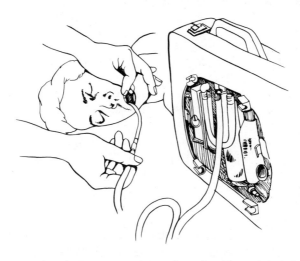

If a patient has been strapped to a long backboard, it is best to simply tip the patient and board to one side.

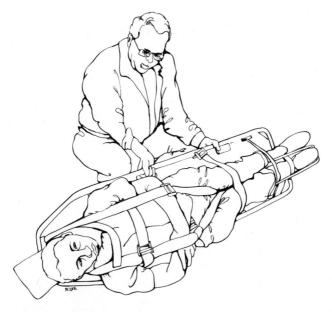

The bag mask ventilator with an oral airway is adequate to ventilate almost any patient, especially when it is necessary to assist the patient's respiration.

The esophageal obturator airway has certain advantages in ventilating a patient who has suffered a *complete cardiopulmonary arrest.* This airway, when properly inserted, will ventilate the patient without distending the stomach with air. The obturator is designed only to prevent gastric contents from rolling into the pharynx, not to stop a patient from vomiting. This point is very important—if a patient vomits with the obturator airway in place, an esophageal laceration could occur. The obturator airway is inserted with the head in the neutral position or slightly anteflexed until the face mask is snug around the mouth. The cuff is distended with air, thereby occluding the esophagus. When air or oxygen is introduced into the opening, it passes down the trachea, ventilating the lungs. After the airway is inserted, the medical technician must listen over both lung fields to ensure that ventilation is adequate and that the airway is not in the trachea.

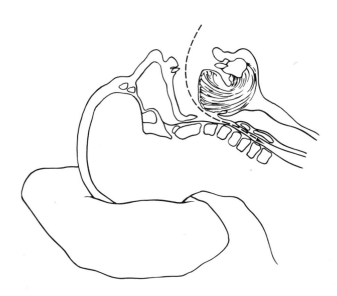

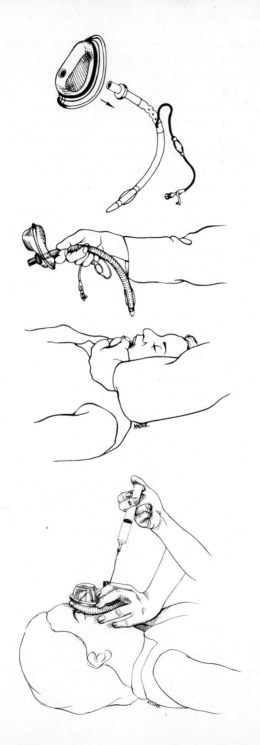

"Cafe Coronary"

It has been suggested that many patients who suffer an apparent myocardial infarction while eating may instead be choking on a bolus of food lodged in the posterior pharynx and obstructing the airway. Although there is presently some controversy surrounding the initial management for these persons, the consensus now is as follows:

1. A patient who is moving air in a limited but adequate manner should be transported to the hospital for definitive management.
2. If the patient is not moving air and cannot speak, in rapid sequence the following course of actions may be followed:
   a. If the patient is prone, mouth-to-mouth ventilation should be attempted to confirm the obstructed airway (see Chap. 2).
   b. Four sharp blows should be delivered between the scapulae in an attempt to dislodge the material.
   c. The Heimlich maneuver may be tried four times with the patient standing or lying.

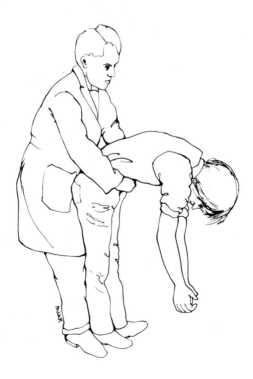

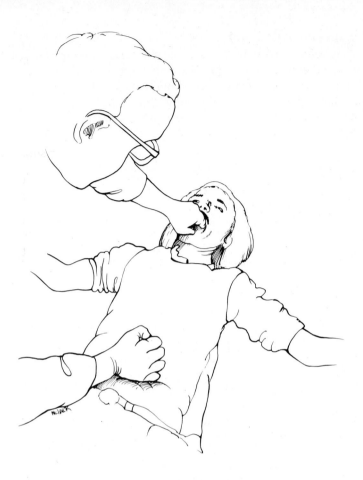

d. Without further delay, cricothyreotomy using a large-bore needle should be performed in an infant or an incision made in an adult (Chap. 8) if the patient's airway is not immediately established by these maneuvers.

2

Cardiopulmonary Resuscitation

Allen P. Klippel

It takes approximately 4 minutes from the moment the heart has ceased to move oxygenated blood until irreversible brain damage occurs. No time can be wasted in looking for equipment or telephoning for help. The patient who has collapsed and has become apneic and whose cyanotic appearance signifies impending death needs nothing more elaborate than immediate restoration of breathing and circulation by the quickest, simplest means. The cause of the ventilatory arrest or cardiac arrest can be sought later. What is needed at that point is immediate institution of assisted ventilation and closed chest cardiac massage.

Respiratory and Cardiac Arrest
SIGNS

1. Increasing cyanosis (unless the patient is very anemic). If the patient has suffered an overdose of a narcotic agent, cyanosis is usually in proportion to the respiratory efforts, which will gradually decrease both in depth and frequency until they stop. The pulse may be slow and bounding.
2. Increased respiratory efforts. Wheezing or "crowing" breath sounds signal upper tract obstruction. Many "heart attacks" in restaurants are due to pharyngeal obstruction by the patient's dentures or a bolus of food. This is especially true in elderly or intoxicated persons.
3. Anoxia is frequently associated with irritable, irrational behavior. Many dying patients fight up to and through their last breath.
4. Mottling of the skin with venous distention and loss of pulse are very late signs—usually too late.

In infant cardiopulmonary resuscitation, the rescuer's mouth is applied over both the infant's mouth and nose. Chest compression of 1 inch over the lower half of the sternum is done with two fingers at a rate of 100 per minute.

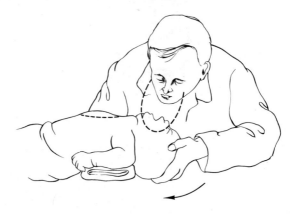

If an oropharyngeal airway of the appropriate size is available, it should be inserted to maintain an open air passage.

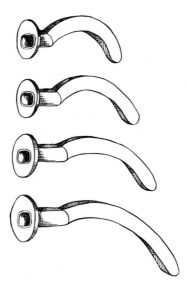

The head is hyperextended, and the airway is inserted over the tongue.

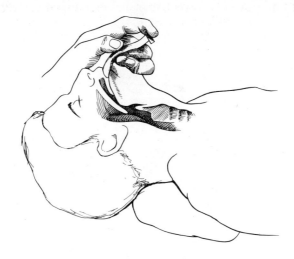

If difficulty is encountered in inserting the airway, it may be inserted from the side and rotated into position.

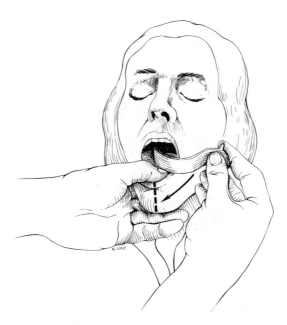

Ventilation can also be assisted by S tubes.

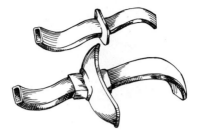

Or pocket mask.

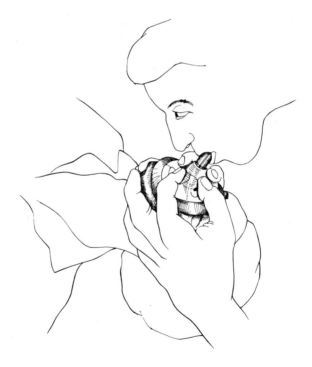

Or bag mask.

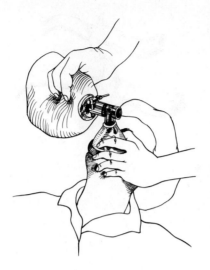

Cardiopulmonary machines powered by oxygen are especially useful in moving patients in situations where ventilation and chest compression would otherwise be interrupted. The oxygen tank is carried on the long backboard between the patient's legs. Pressure-cycled respirators (inhalators) are not recommended, since they are ineffective if any degree of airway obstruction is present.

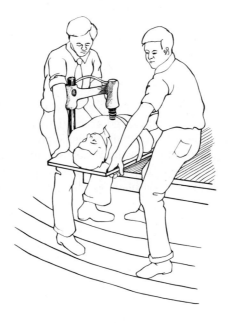

ENDOTRACHEAL INTUBATION IN CARDIAC ARREST
Endotracheal intubation must be done only by experts who require only a few seconds to insert the tube. Usually a 6.5- to 7-mm tube is used in a woman and a 7.5- to 8-mm tube in a man. For infants, use a tube of a size that will fit the infant's external nasal opening.

The head is hyperextended. It may be helpful to put a folded towel under the patient's occiput.

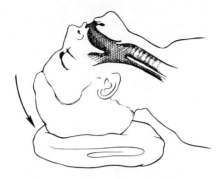

The laryngoscope must not lever against the teeth. It should be held in the left hand, introduced at the right side of the mouth, and thrust 45° upward to raise the tongue and floor of the mouth and put the head and neck into the "sniffing" position. The epiglottis is visualized, and if a straight-blade laryngoscope is used the tip of the straight-blade is placed over the epiglottis to expose the cords.

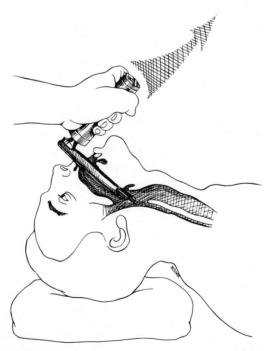

The tip of the curved-blade laryngoscope (Macintosh) is inserted between the base of the tongue and the epiglottis to visualize the larynx.

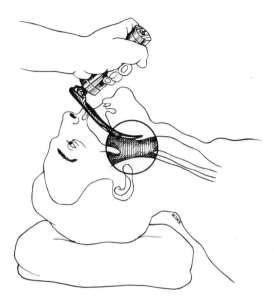

The vocal cords must be clearly visualized, and the tube must be seen to pass between them.

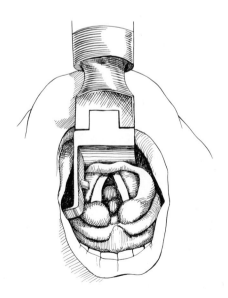

After the endotracheal tube has been inserted, the cuff is inflated. Low-pressure cuffed tubes are preferred. Low-pressure tubes with two cuffs that can be alternately inflated to avoid tracheal ulcers are especially important when it is expected that respiratory assistance will be necessary for a prolonged period. It is mandatory that auscultation be done over both lung fields to ensure that the tube is in the trachea and that ventilation is occurring.

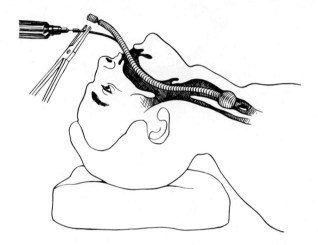

If an esophageal obturator airway has previously been inserted, leave it in place until the endotracheal tube is in place and inflated. Otherwise, the gastric contents may roll into the pharynx and obstruct the view of the larynx, or be aspirated into the trachea, or both.

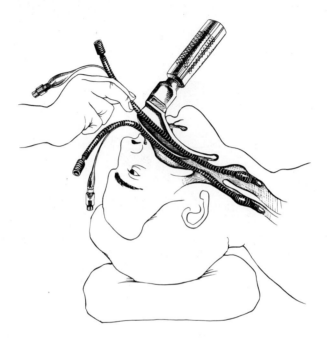

After the patient is well ventilated and while the circulation is being maintained by closed chest massage, preparation for electric cardioversion or defibrillation is made. One defibrillator paddle is placed just caudal to the right clavicle at the right sternal border and the other paddle on the left chest caudal to the left breast or pectoral muscle. The usual current used is 400 watt-seconds.

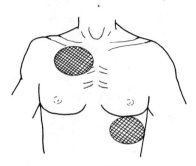

Defibrillator paddle positions

It is beyond the scope of this book to enumerate all of the techniques and drugs involved in cardiac resuscitation except to suggest that the protocol be followed that is advocated by the American Heart Association for Advanced Cardiac Life Support.

Open Chest Cardiac Compression
INDICATIONS

1. In cardiac arrest following cardiac tamponade, but only if aspiration has not been successful.
2. In tension pneumothorax, with the heart displaced laterally.
3. In a markedly emphysematous patient with a rigid, hyperexpanded chest that cannot be compressed.
4. In a patient who has suffered exsanguination, with a heart so small as to preclude closed chest massage.
5. In a patient with a displaced heart (pectus excavatum).

PROCEDURE
The incision is made through the fourth interspace (under the left breast), from the sternum to the posterior rib cage. Avoid or ligate the internal thoracic artery after the patient's circulation has been restored. The incision should be made through the skin and muscles simultaneously.

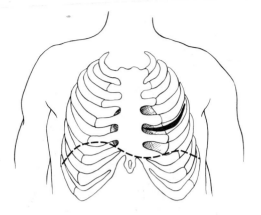

Open the interspace and insert a rib spreader if available.

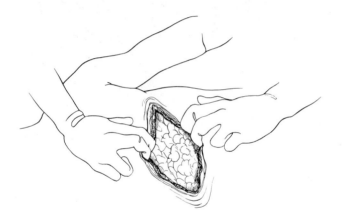

Open the pericardial sac, avoiding the phrenic nerve, which lies on the posterior lateral aspect of the pericardium.

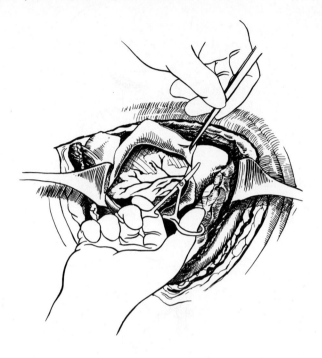

Compress the ventricles of the heart by pushing from behind
against the sternum with one hand.

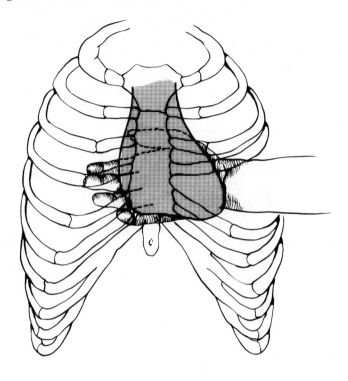

Compression of small hearts may be done by using only the right hand, which squeezes the ventricles between the fingers posteriorly and the palm of the hand (thenar eminence) anteriorly. Squeeze with the flat of the fingers, not the fingertips, which could perforate the weakened myocardium.

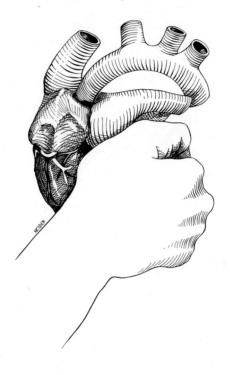

Large hearts may have to be compressed with the palm of one hand anteriorly and the fingers of the other hand posteriorly.

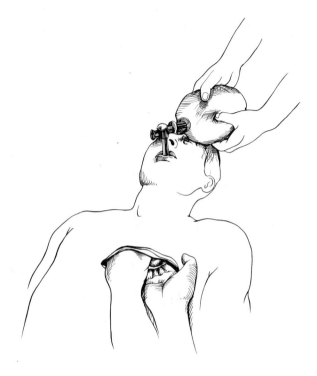

Internal defibrillation is accomplished by applying paddle electrodes with saline-soaked pads to the exposed ventricles. One paddle is applied to the anterior surface of the heart and another to the posterior surface of the left ventricle; 50 watt-seconds of direct current countershock is used.

Transthoracic Pacing (Temporary)

This procedure is not as satisfactory as inserting a transvenous pacemaker, but it may be considered in some emergency situations. The equipment is packaged already sterilized by manufacturers. The patient must be on a monitor.

Under sterile conditions the left chest is prepared and draped. The needle is inserted through the skin of the fourth interspace 2 cm to the left of the sternal border. The obturator is removed, and blood should escape or be drawn by the syringe, confirming placement in the ventricle. The pacing wire is inserted through the needle, and the needle is then removed. The terminals are connected to the power source. Considerable care must be taken to ensure that each terminal is inserted into the proper location on the connector to the power source. The electrode wire is withdrawn gently until it offers resistance, indicating it is caught against the wall of the ventricle. A single suture is placed around the catheter and tied to hold it in place.

Pacing is started at 5 milliamperes, at a rate of 75 per minute. If capture is achieved, the milliampere output is reduced to the least amount that allows for continuing pacing. A permanent or transvenous pacemaker should be inserted as soon as possible.

Transthoracic pacing may also be performed by inserting the needle from the subxiphoid position. This area is prepared and draped, and the needle is inserted along the left side of the xiphoid, pointed toward the midpoint of the clavicle. Otherwise, the technique is similar to that described above for inserting the pacemaker through the anterior chest.

Insertion of a Temporary Transvenous Pacemaker

The technique for inserting a temporary transvenous pacemaker is similar to that used for a venous cutdown. The patient must be on a cardiac monitor to watch for arrhythmias as well as to document capture by the pacemaker. Pacing of the heart is a difficult task and not without danger and should be done by physicians experienced in the technique and under fluoroscopic observation when possible. If the catheter does not seat properly in the apex of the ventricle, it will not pace properly. There is also a considerable risk of penetrating the ventricle.

INDICATIONS
1. Complete heart block with episodes of:
   a. Asystole.
   b. Ventricular bradycardia.
2. Complete heart block following myocardial infarction.
3. Mobitz type II block (standby pacemaker).
4. Sinus bradycardia with Stokes-Adams syndrome.
5. Cardiac arrest with asystole.

PROCEDURE
A 2-cm transverse incision is made over the basilic vein of the right arm cephalad to the cubital space after routine preparation and draping has been done.

After the vein is exposed, a 4-0 chromic catgut tie is placed behind the proximal portion and held. Another catgut tie is passed behind the distal portion of the vein, and this ligature is tied around the vessel.

A small opening is made in the vein, and the bipolar electrode is inserted and advanced into the left ventricle. This is best done observing the catheter under the fluoroscope to ensure that it is properly located at the apex and in a stable position. The positive and negative terminals of the catheter are then connected to the power source, which is started at 5 milliamperes of current and usually at 70 to 75 beats per minute.

After capture of the heart has been achieved, the proximal ligature is tied around the vein and catheter. The power output is reduced to the lowest that continues to capture.

The skin incision is closed with interrupted silk sutures. One of these sutures is also tied around the catheter. Antibiotic ointment is applied at the skin opening, and a sterile dressing is applied.

If a fluoroscope is not available, the power source is attached to the electrode, which is advanced until it is calculated that the tip is in the right atrium of the heart. The power is set at 5 milliamperes with a rate of 75 beats per minute. While the electrocardiograph is watched, the electrode is advanced into the ventricle until capture of the heart has been achieved. Again, if capture is achieved, the output is reduced to the lowest compatible with continuing cardiac capture.

Insertion of a Swan-Ganz Catheter

Measurement of the pulmonary wedge pressure is essential in the management of patients in shock states resulting from various conditions, especially following myocardial infarction or during resuscitation with large amounts of blood or other fluids.

The pulmonary venous pressure reflects the level of pulmonary congestion and the pressure in the left atrium. If there is no mitral valvular disease, it may also approximate the left ventricular diastolic pressure, provided that level is below 15 mm Hg. In a patient with myocardial infarction the wedge pressure can indicate whether the patient is suffering from pump failure or from hypovolemia in addition to the myocardial injury. In the former, the pressure will be elevated, indicating the need for inotropic agents; in hypovolemic shock, the pressure will be low.

Cardiac output can also be measured using thermodilution techniques if the catheter is fitted with a thermistor.

TECHNIQUE

The patient must be on a cardiac monitor to watch for arrhythmias. If the vein is large, percutaneous insertion may be possible with a large-bore needle that is removed after the catheter is started.

A 2-cm incision is made over the left basilic vein proximal to the cubital space. The vein is isolated, and two 4-0 catgut ties are passed behind. The distal ligature is tied. A small opening is made in the vein. The catheter, usually a No. 5 balloon flotation type, is connected to the pressure monitor and advanced. In the average patient the catheter will advance 45 to 50 cm from the left cubital space, 35 to 40 cm from the right cubital fossa, and 10 to 15 cm from internal jugular or subclavian sites.

When the catheter is in the thorax, the pressure will be seen to vary with respiration. At this point the balloon is inflated with air to the recommended amount. The pressures and wave forms obtained in the right atrium, right ventricle, and pulmonary artery are noted. The pressure in the right atrium is about 5 mm Hg, with shallow undulations. In the right ventricle the pressure wave increases sharply in amplitude. As the pulmonary artery is entered, the systolic value remains about the same as in the ventricle, but the diastolic value rises to 15 to 25 mm Hg. When the catheter wedges, the fluctuations are dampened at approximately the same value as the ventricular diastolic reading, so that the reading becomes almost a straight line. The balloon is then deflated, which allows the catheter to return to the pulmonary artery, as indicated by alternating systolic and diastolic pressures.

Measurements must not be made constantly, but only every 15 to 30 minutes. When the balloon is to be reinflated, a bolus of 0.2 ml of air is injected and pressures observed and this procedure repeated until a single diastolic pressure is maintained, indicating wedging. If wedging is observed at considerably less than the recommended filling, the catheter must be withdrawn 1 to 2 cm, since it may be in a small artery and could act as an embolus.

When it is judged that the catheter is in satisfactory position, the proximal ligature is tied around the vein and the catheter. The skin incision is closed with interrupted nonabsorbable sutures, one of which may also be tied around the catheter. An antibiotic ointment and a dry dressing are then placed on the wound.

3

Vascular Catheterizations

Charles B. Anderson

Expeditious percutaneous cannulation of veins and arteries is essential for the proper management of critically ill patients. A cutdown may be necessary for intravenous infusions if vessels can not be palpated or identified by surface landmarks. If arterial blood samples will be required frequently over a period of several days, a radial artery cutdown may be preferred to repeated arterial needle sticks. The blood pressure can also be monitored by a radial artery catheter. Percutaneous needle cannulation will suffice for most emergency situations. Shaving the skin is not required for needle cannulation, but should be completed prior to performing a cutdown. The area is prepared with an antiseptic solution, with special care taken if blood cultures are to be obtained.

The size of the syringe will depend on the amount of blood needed. When drawing arterial blood samples for blood gas determinations, 3- to 5-ml syringes are used; 10- to 30-ml syringes are used to draw venous blood for general testing.

For aspirating venous blood, 19-, 20-, 21-gauge needles are used; 23- or 25-gauge needles are used for arterial blood sampling because they leave a smaller hole in the vessel wall, which seals better under arterial pressure than a hole made by a larger-gauge needle.

Complications following vascular catheterization include infection, thrombosis of the vessel, hemorrhage into the surrounding soft tissue, or external bleeding if a sealed tract is not present. Pressure should be applied for several minutes in the case of venous punctures and 5 to 10 minutes with arterial punctures. Following arterial puncture, the site should be inspected after 30 minutes to ensure that hemostasis has occurred.

Several types of needles are available for venous cannulations: straight needles, scalpel-vein needles with "butterfly wings," intracath needles in which the tubing passes through the needle, and Medicut catheters in which the metal needle fits inside the catheter. Plastic tubing of various sizes that must be adapted with a blunt tipped needle is also available for cutdown cannulation when the vein is exposed and surgically opened.

Venipuncture

Venous blood for routine laboratory studies is usually obtained from veins in the antecubital fossa, the radial aspect of the wrist (cephalic vein), or the dorsum of the hand. Localization of the appropriate vein may require palpation rather than direct visualization. It is often easier to feel than to see a compressibly soft distended vein when there is venous hypertension from a tourniquet placed around the upper arm.

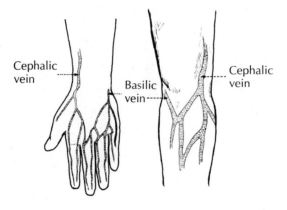

Secondary choices for venipuncture include the external jugular vein in the neck, the femoral vein in the groin, and, less frequently, the veins of the foot. Needle aspiration of blood from the femoral vein is contraindicated in patients with pulmonary emboli because of the possibility of dislodging clots from the vessel wall and subsequent central embolization. In infants, heel sticks can provide enough blood to perform blood analyses by microtechniques.

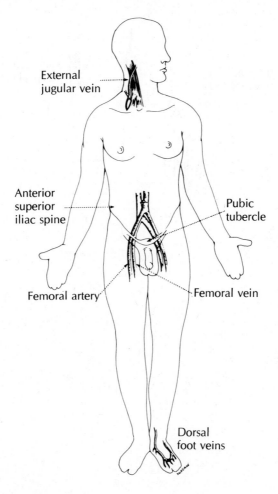

External
jugular vein

Anterior
superior
iliac spine

Pubic
tubercle

Femoral artery

Femoral vein

Dorsal
foot veins

The arrangement of veins in the antecubital fossa is variable, but in general medial (basilic) and lateral (cephalic) veins with a median cubital vein joining the two will be encountered. Aspiration of blood from the antecubital fossa veins begins with the placement of a tourniquet around the upper portion of the arm sufficiently tight to prevent venous return yet permit arterial inflow. The arm is supinated and kept in a dependent position. The patient opens and closes his hand for a half a minute to aid venous distention. The antecubital fossa is lightly slapped or briskly rubbed to raise the veins. In difficult situations the veins may be dilated by applying a hot, wet towel for 5 to 10 minutes. The area is wiped with alcohol, and the needle is then inserted obliquely at a 45° angle under the skin for a distance of 3 to 4 mm. The vein is pierced, and if a vacuum tube is used, it will start filling.

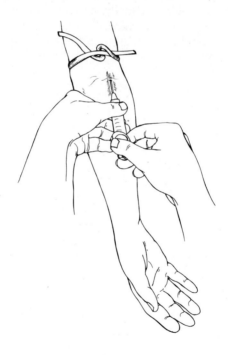

By inserting the needle obliquely, a subcutaneous tract is formed that will help seal the venous puncture site when the needle is withdrawn.

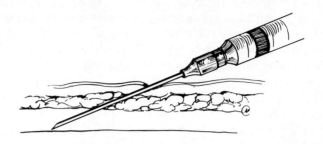

The syringe is gently aspirated to obtain blood. If blood is not forthcoming, the needle is withdrawn or advanced slightly until the vein lumen is entered. Usually, a slight popping sensation is felt when the vein wall is pierced. During withdrawal of blood, the tourniquet should be released and the arm kept in the dependent position.

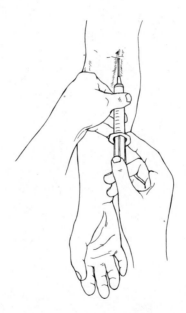

The needle is withdrawn and pressure applied by the patient over the puncture site for several minutes.

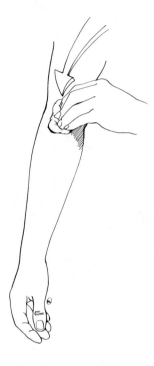

The use of vacuum tubes for venous blood sampling can greatly facilitate and speed the process. A variety of vacuum tubes contain different anticoagulants (depending on the test), or no anticoagulant if serum is desired. The rubber stoppers are color coded to indicate the type of anticoagulant present. A chart or list is available outlining the applicable code system.

The apparatus is assembled by screwing the double-ended needle (short needle end) into one end of the adapter.

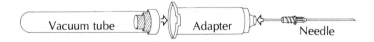

Vacuum tube   Adapter   Needle

The vacuum tube is put into the other end of the adapter, and the tube is pushed forward so that the short needle enters the rubber stopper but does not pierce it completely; thus the vacuum remains intact.

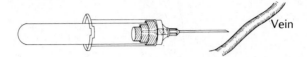

Once the vein is entered, the vacuum is broken by advancing the tube further. Blood then is sucked into the tube.

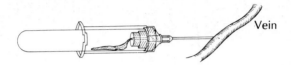

Multiple tubes may be filled simply by exchanging them as the needle, with adapter attached, is held securely within the vein lumen.

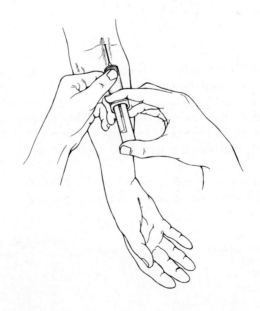

In children and adults, the external jugular vein can be used. The patient is placed in the Trendelenburg position. The head is down and pressure is applied at the base of the neck to cause distention of the vein that crosses the sternocleidomastoid muscle. The head is turned to the opposite side. Cannulation of the vein and aspiration of blood is then completed.

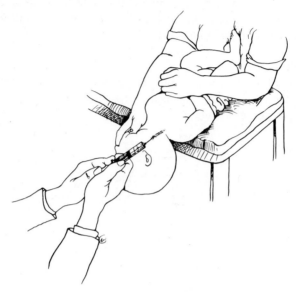

The femoral vein can also be used when other sites are not available. The vein lies just medial to the artery below the inguinal ligament. The femoral artery pulse is felt in the groin. A needle with attached syringe is inserted perpendicular to the skin 0.5 to 1.0 cm medial to the artery and 2 cm below the inguinal ligament. The needle is advanced while gentle aspiration is maintained on the syringe. Blood will be obtained as the needle tip enters the vein lumen. If the needle is inserted quickly, it may penetrate the front *and* back walls of the vein, reaching the pubic ramus. Maintaining suction, the needle should be withdrawn slowly back into the vein lumen. Care should be taken to avoid the femoral artery. If the artery is inadvertently punctured and a good flow obtained, the blood sample may be obtained from this vessel and prolonged (10 minutes) pressure applied after the needle is removed. More commonly, a hematoma starts to form because the needle is not lying properly inside the arterial lumen. In this case, the needle should be withdrawn, pressure applied, and the opposite groin used for the venous sample.

Venous Cannulation

PERCUTANEOUS CANNULATION

Most veins used for aspiration of venous blood are also suitable for percutaneous cannulation with plastic catheters. Flexion creases should be avoided because movement may dislodge the needle or catheter. After a needle or catheter has been secured in position, a topical antibiotic ointment should be applied to the skin puncture site and meticulous care taken to prevent initial and subsequent contamination.

Butterflies

Insertion of a small ¾-inch butterfly-type needle into a forearm vein is the simplest approach. It is taped into position and covered by a sterile dressing.

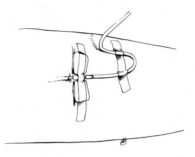

Intracath

Portions of the intracath are enclosed in a cellophane envelope that permits handling without contamination (A). The envelope, the metal obturator, the cannula, the needle, and the plastic shield constitute the separate parts (B).

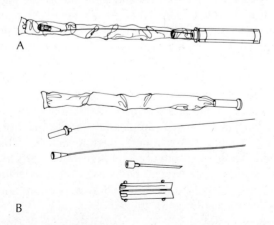

A

B

Almost any vein can be cannulated with the use of an intracath because the catheter tip can be placed at different locations and movements of joints will not result in dislodgment. The vein is punctured and the needle set securely inside the vein.

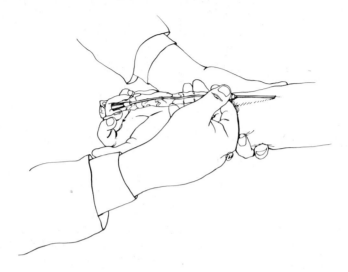

The catheter is advanced into the vein by manipulation through the cellophane envelope. An inner wire stent is usually withdrawn slightly to facilitate advancement of the plastic catheter. The catheter is advanced completely until the hub of the needle is reached and the catheter end firmly joined to it.

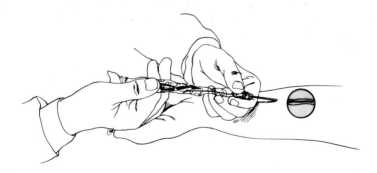

The cellophane envelope is removed by twisting it slightly at the hub while the needle and catheter are held securely.

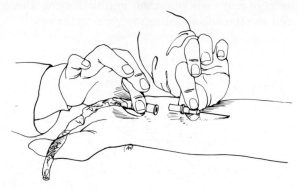

The wire stent is removed.

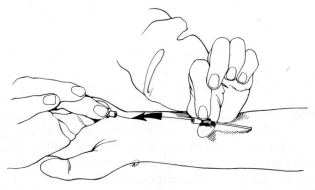

The needle, along with the catheter, is withdrawn slightly and the plastic shield slipped into position. The tip of the needle is splinted to prevent cutting the catheter.

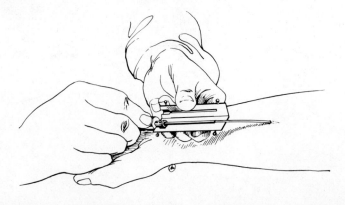

Intravenous tubing is connected to the catheter, and the tubing and catheter are securely taped to the forearm. The plastic catheter should never be pulled back through the needle, since it can be sheared off by the sharp needle point, with subsequent embolization to the right side of the heart. Antibiotic ointment is applied to the skin puncture site before placing the dressing.

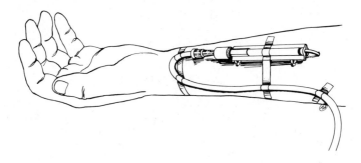

Medicut
Components of the Medicut catheter are in a sterile container (1). The entire apparatus, when connected (2), consists of a firm plastic catheter placed over a needle that is connected to a syringe (3).

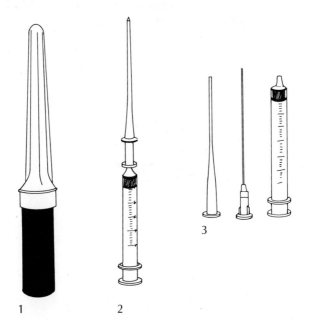

The stiff Medicut does not bend easily and should not be inserted across joints. The forearm is steadied and punctured with the assembled Medicut apparatus.

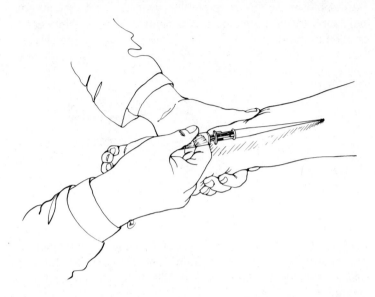

The syringe is aspirated and blood withdrawn, confirming that the vein lumen has been entered.

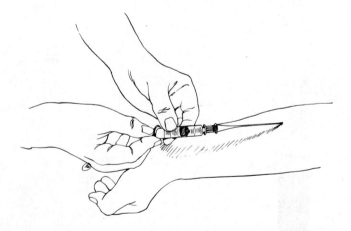

The plastic Medicut catheter is then advanced over the needle further into the vein, and the needle and syringe are withdrawn.

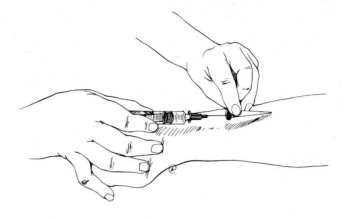

Intravenous tubing is connected to the catheter, which is taped in place.

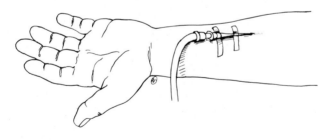

VENOUS CUTDOWN

Skin incisions with direct visualization of the vein is performed when percutaneous catheterization is not possible, or when large catheters must be inserted.

Any adequately sized vein may be used, but preferred sites include the following: the cephalic vein in the deltopectoral groove of the shoulder; the external jugular vein in the neck; the saphenous vein in the groin; the saphenous vein anterior to the medial maleolus in the ankle; or any large vein in the arm, forearm, or wrist. The consistent location of the saphenous vein in the ankle makes this a preferred site when emergency vascular access is essential, since the vein can be quickly identified.

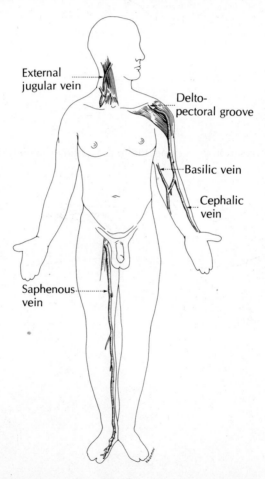

External jugular vein

Delto-pectoral groove

Basilic vein

Cephalic vein

Saphenous vein

After preparing and draping, a 3-cm transverse skin incision is made anterior to the medial maleolus.

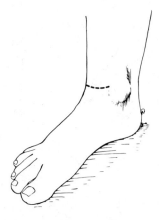

With blunt dissection, a clamp is placed deep into the wound and passed from a medial to lateral position, keeping close to the bone. This maneuver will pick up the saphenous vein. Fatty areolar tissue is separated from around the vein.

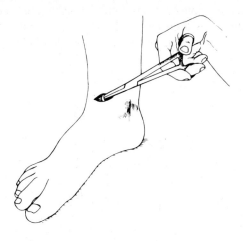

The vein is ligated distally, controlled proximally with a loop of silk suture, and partially incised with a scissors between the two silk sutures.

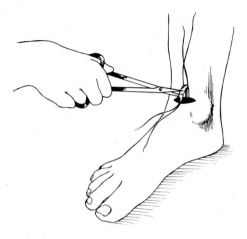

A plastic catheter is inserted into the vein, directed proximally, and tied into position with the two silk sutures. The catheter is brought out through a separate stab wound, and the incision is closed with interrupted sutures. Intravenous tubing is connected, and the catheter is then taped in place. A separate skin suture surrounding the plastic catheter will prevent accidental dislodgment.

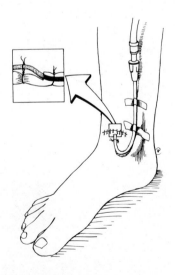

Subclavian Catheterization

The subclavian vein lying under the clavicle is a readily accessible vessel that can accommodate a large catheter for rapid intravenous infusions or central venous pressure monitoring. Once the catheter is inserted, it is located away from any joint movement. The catheter can be left for prolonged periods if proper antiseptic techniques are used at the time of insertion and wound care is meticulous.

Complications of this procedure include pneumothorax from trauma to the lung in the apex of the pleural space, hematoma formation from subclavian artery penetration, a combined hemopneumothorax, and sepsis from a contaminated catheter. If the patient has a pulmonary problem such as pneumonia or pneumothorax, the side *with* the disease should be chosen for subclavian vein cannulation. Should insertion of the catheter on the side opposite the lesion result in a complication (e.g., pneumothorax) the patient's respiratory status would be severely compromised because of the reduction in effective ventilation in the normal side.

The patient is placed in the Trendelenburg position, to permit dilation of the vein, and the shoulders are hyperextended over a rolled towel placed along the thoracic spine. The shoulders are depressed downward and the head turned to the opposite side. The skin over the lower neck, shoulder, and chest is carefully shaved and prepared with antiseptic solution. Strict aseptic technique is used, with appropriate draping and the use of sterile gloves.

An assistant places a finger in the suprasternal notch to direct passage of the needle. The midportion of the clavicle is identified by palpation. Just caudal to the midportion of the clavicle, a skin wheal is raised by the injection of local anesthesia. A 14-gauge intracath needle is inserted in a horizontal plane and is directed toward the finger in the suprasternal notch.

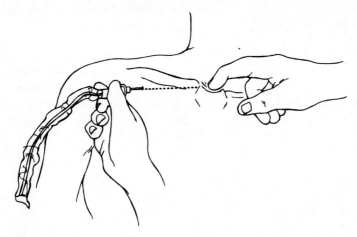

The subclavian vein lies anterior to the artery and crosses over the first rib. The needle is inserted in a direction that conforms to that of the vein. An alternative method involves the attachment of a 10-ml syringe to the 14-gauge needle to maintain slight gentle suction as the needle is advanced. A closed system is maintained to prevent air embolism should the patient inspire deeply. The patient is instructed to hold his breath during the brief periods when the intracath tube is advanced through the open needle or the intravenous tubing is being connected.

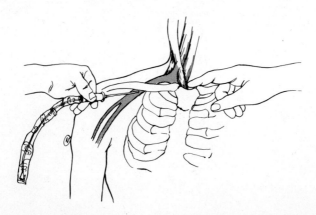

When the vein is entered, blood will appear in the intracath tubing or in the aspirating syringe. The operator then advances the intracath tubing, being sure to remove the wired stent slightly so that only the tip of the intracath abuts against the internal surface of the vein. If a syringe is used, it must be detached and a sterile catheter inserted through the needle.

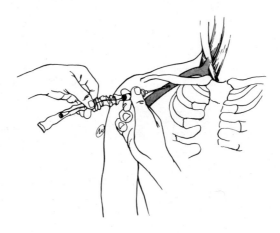

The catheter is advanced until it lies in the superior vena cava. The distance may be judged by using the metal stent. If the catheter is advanced too far, it will lie in the right ventricle, and excessive pulsatile pressures will be recorded. If the catheter is inserted too far across the tricuspid valve into the right ventricle, arrhythmias may be induced. Finally, the catheter is sutured to the skin, antibiotic ointment placed about the skin puncture site, and a dressing applied.

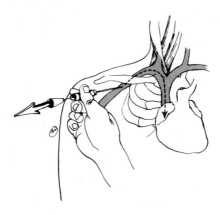

An upright chest roentgenogram is obtained to be sure that a pneumothorax has not been produced and that the radiopaque catheter is properly positioned.

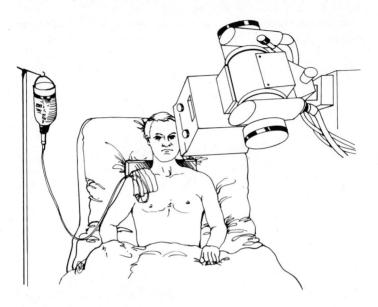

Internal Jugular Vein Catheterization

Cannulation of the internal jugular vein is an alternate method to subclavian vein catheterization; it can be used for central venous pressure monitoring and maintenance of a large-bore catheter for venous access.

With the patient in the Trendelenburg position, the 14-gauge needle with attached syringe is directed into the internal jugular vein via an approach between the two heads of the sterno-cleidomastoid muscle that inserts into the sternum and clavicle.

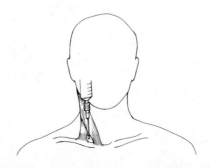

This approach involves piercing the skin at the apex of the triangle formed by the two heads of the sternocleidomastoid muscle and directing the needle inferiorly and posteriorly at a 30° angle to the skin. It is important to keep the needle parallel to the midline to avoid the carotid artery. When blood is aspirated, the patient is told to hold his breath, the syringe is removed, and the catheter is threaded into the superior vena cava. The intra-cath needle is then pulled back, the intravenous tubing connected, the catheter sutured to the skin, antibiotic ointment applied, and a dressing secured.

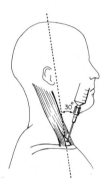

Arterial Cannulations

The radial, brachial, and femoral arteries are used to obtain arterial blood samples for pH and blood gas analysis. The femoral artery is easiest to cannulate, but has a greater risk of serious vascular complications than do the others. The radial artery is the most difficult to cannulate, but trauma to this vessel is usually not important. The Allen test should always be performed prior to any needle aspiration of blood from the radial artery and certainly before long-term cannulation of this vessel, which often requires distal ligation and the potential of radial artery thrombosis. If there is inadequate ulnar artery collateral blood supply to the hand, radial artery obstruction might result in an insufficient vascular supply to the hand.

The Allen test is performed by digital occlusion of both the radial and ulnar arteries while the patient forcefully closes his hand to empty it of blood. When release of pressure on one of the arteries is immediately followed by flushing of the hand, an adequate blood supply to the hand from that artery is indicated. Absence of a flush on release of the ulnar artery indicates that the main blood supply to that hand is via the radial artery and that trauma to this vessel should be avoided.

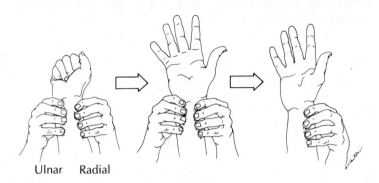

Ulnar   Radial

A 25-gauge, 1½ inch needle is attached to a 3-ml syringe. The syringe is coated with heparin solution (1,000 units per milliliter) by aspirating the heparin into the syringe. For arterial blood gas determinations, each milliliter of blood should be mixed with 0.05 ml of heparin (1,000 units per milliliter). Greater amounts of heparin will cause the pH to be falsely acidotic, and lesser amounts may be inadequate for anticoagulation.

RADIAL ARTERY

The hand is supinated and hyperextended over a towel, exposing the flexor surface of the wrist. Anesthesia is not necessary. The radial artery is palpated and a 23- or 25-gauge needle inserted at a 45° angle over the artery, just distal to the fingers. When pulsations from the arterial wall are felt, the needle is quickly thrust forward into the lumen. Usually, the posterior arterial wall is pierced, and the needle must be slightly withdrawn for the needle tip to lie within the vessel lumen. After aspirating 2 to 3 ml of blood, the needle is removed and pressure is maintained for 5 minutes.

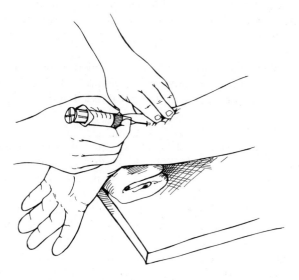

A slight modification involves the use of a 25-gauge needle without the attached syringe. When the artery is properly taped, a strong pulsatile flow of blood occurs and the syringe can then be connected. This method incurs minimal pain and reduces the chances of obtaining venous blood.

The radial artery is the artery most commonly used for continuous pressure monitoring. It can be cannulated percutaneously using a Medicut catheter or performing a cutdown to locate the vessel more accurately.

Radial artery cannulation by a cutdown technique will be necessary when repeated arterial blood samples are needed or continuous accurate monitoring of blood pressure is required.

The wrist area is prepared, draped, and infiltrated with local anesthesia. A transverse skin incision is made just proximal to the flexion crease at the wrist, and the flexor retinaculum is identified and divided longitudinally over the radial artery. The artery is mobilized and the distal end tied with a 2-0 silk ligature; the proximal side is controlled with another silk ligature looped around the artery. A transverse incision is made in the artery, a catheter inserted, and the proximal ligature tied. The distal ligature is tied around the catheter to prevent its dislodgment, and the catheter is brought out through the incision or a separate stab wound. The incision is closed with interrupted sutures, and intravenous tubing is secured to the catheter. A three-way stopcock and heparinized saline solution are used to keep the line from clotting.

An alternate method involves the cannulation of the radial artery with a Medicut catheter after first surgically exposing the vessel. This avoids suture ligation of the distal radial artery.

BRACHIAL ARTERY

The brachial artery is identified at the medial aspect of the antecubetal fossa. The median nerve crosses from lateral to medial underneath the artery, but is usually not disturbed by the procedure. The forearm is supinated, and the artery is immobilized between two fingers of one hand. When the artery is fixed, the needle is placed through the skin toward the artery. The needle is inserted at a 45° to 90° angle to the skin. As the surface of the artery is encountered and pulsations are felt, the needle is quickly advanced by thrusting it into the artery. The needle should not be advanced too far or it will exit through the posterior wall. With gentle suction and withdrawal of the needle the arterial lumen will be encountered and blood obtained. With systolic blood pressures greater than 100 mm Hg, the syringe usually self-fills, and aspiration is not necessary. Filling confirms that an artery has been entered. After the needle is removed, pressure is applied for 5 to 10 minutes.

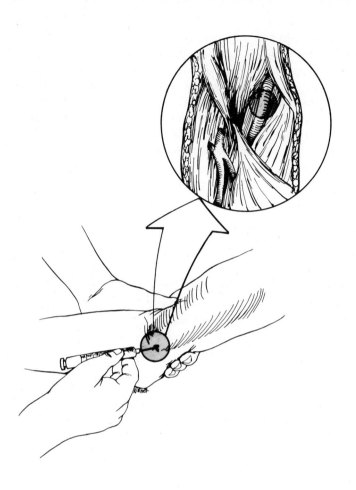

FEMORAL ARTERY

The femoral artery is fixed longitudinally between the index and third fingers of one hand. The area selected is approximately 2 cm below the inguinal ligament. The aspirating syringe and needle are inserted perpendicular to the skin until the surface of the femoral artery is identified by pulsations transmitted through the needle. The needle is quickly thrust forward as if one were throwing a dart, and the wall of the artery is pierced.

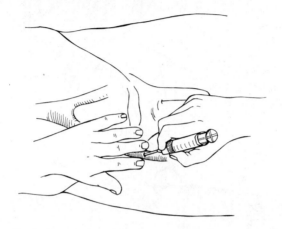

If the needle has passed through both the anterior and posterial walls of the artery, initial aspiration will not result in obtaining blood.

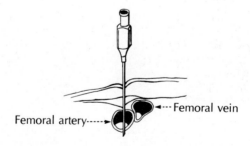

Femoral artery----► ◄--- Femoral vein

However, as the needle is withdrawn, the vascular lumen is entered and arterial blood flows into the syringe. To be sure that the femoral artery has been entered, the syringe is temporarily removed and a pulsatile flow of blood demonstrated. Spontaneous filling of the syringe without aspirating also indicates that the needle lies in an arterial lumen.

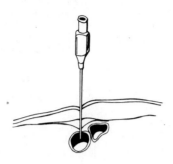

4

Basic Surgical Techniques

Charles B. Anderson

Familiarization with basic surgical instruments and the correct methods of using them is essential for the proper management of either iatrogenic or traumatic wounds. Selection of the proper needle and suture material will enhance the final operative result. Ability to tie knots quickly and accurately either by hand or instrument is important. Certain basic principles can be applied to the preparation, initial management, and closure of most wounds.

Instruments

Most surgical problems can be managed in the emergency department with just a few surgical instruments from among the wide variety available.

SCALPEL AND BLADES

A No. 3 scalpel handle can accommodate several different medium-sized blades. Number 10 blades are used for routine dissection; No. 15 blades are used for fine dissection of smaller structures. A No. 11 blade is pointed and is used for incising hollow structures such as abscesses. For fine dissection the scalpel is grasped like a pencil with the wrist supported on a firm, flat surface. To make the initial skin incision the scalpel is grasped between the thumb and middle fingers, with the index finger used to steady the top of the blade. Hard structures such as steel or bone will dull the blade after a single stroke.

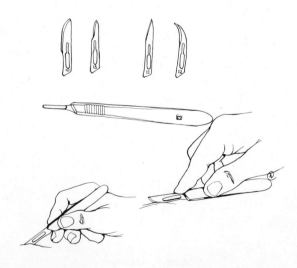

To incise an abscess, the blade is inserted so that the cutting edge faces upward and is directed outward to avoid accidental damage of deeper structures. A No. 12 hooked blade can also be used in a similar manner.

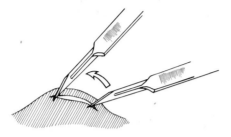

The blade should be held with a hemostat forceps rather than the fingers when inserted into or removed from the scalpel handle to prevent accidental cutting of the surgeon. Each blade fits the handle in only one manner because the blade is beveled and conforms to the angle at the neck of the handle.

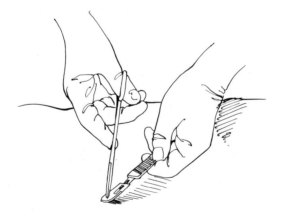

Blades are removed by grasping with a hemostat, elevating the base of the blade and sliding it off the end of the scalpel.

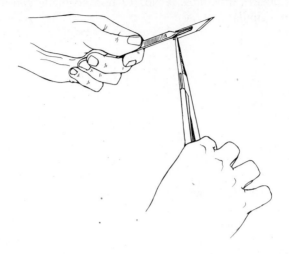

FORCEPS

Tissue forceps have teeth that hold firmly and prevent slipping. These forceps should never be used when blood vessels, bowel, or other delicate structures are handled. Limited pressure is required, because the teeth prevent slippage. A variety of sizes is available. Thumb forceps without teeth are used when dissecting tissue that should not be perforated. They are never used on skin because excessive pressure is required to obtain a firm grasp, and pressure necrosis of the skin would result. Fine tooth forceps are used during closure of the skin, because the small perforations permit the skin to be held firmly with minimal pressure. Most forceps are held between the thumb and the index and middle fingers and are usually placed in the nondominant hand to free the opposite hand for dissection.

Forceps as well as other instruments can be palmed with the fourth and fifth fingers to free the remaining fingers for holding and using other instruments. This maneuver speeds surgical procedures because instruments do not have to be passed back and forth.

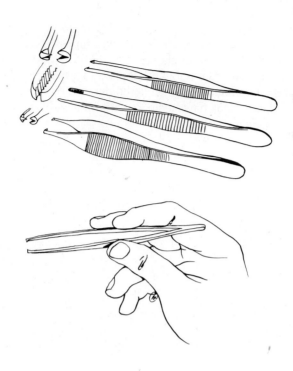

CLAMPS

Clamps are available in many sizes and shapes. Straight arterial clamps and curved Kelly clamps are used to control medium-sized vessels. They are held and applied in a manner similar to that used when handling a needle holder (see Needle Holders). Kocher clamps that have teeth on the end are used to place traction on heavy fascia.

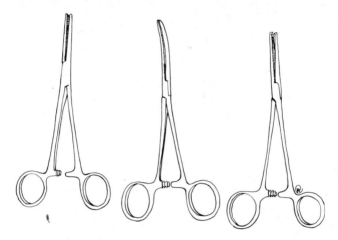

Fine mosquito forceps, both curved (left) and straight (middle), are used to control bleeding from small, delicate vessels. These clamps will tear loose if undue traction is applied. An Allis clamp has small, serrated teeth and is used to grasp fascia or other structures such as cysts, which must be manipulated to facilitate exposure and dissection. It is not applied to the skin because of crushing necrosis.

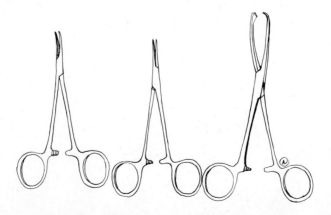

TOWEL CLIPS

The towel clip, which has two sharp, pointed tips, holds the edges of the drapes in place. The clip can pass through the skin to obtain a firm anchorage; anesthesia of the skin is obviously required. The instrument can also be used to grasp the skin for traction purposes.

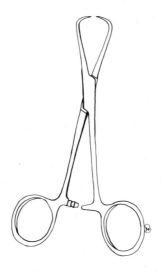

DISSECTING SCISSORS

Metzenbaum scissors (left) are light, fine scissors used for general tissue dissection. They have a slight curve to the tip. The heavier and shorter Mayo scissors (center) are used for cutting tough fascia. Sharp pointed dissecting scissors (right) are used where delicate small structures are encountered. Although scissors are held in a variety of ways, they are most often grasped with the thumb and fourth fingers inserted through the rings, with the index finger placed to steady the instrument. Dissecting scissors should never be used to cut sutures, since this will dull and malalign the blades.

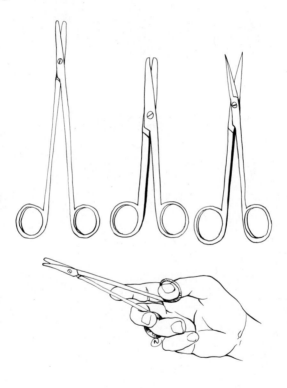

SUTURE AND BANDAGE SCISSORS

Straight, heavy suture scissors are used to cut most suture material except wire. The tips are blunt, to avoid inadvertent trauma. Suture scissors are steadied with the opposite hand while the material is cut under good visualization.

Suture removal scissors have a hooked tip that can be inserted under the skin suture. The sutures often become taut in edematous skin and are hard to elevate without the hooked tip. Bandage scissors have one sharp blade tip, and the other blunt and rounded. The blunt blade is inserted under the bandage. This pushes away the skin as the blunt tip is advanced. Bandage scissors are well constructed to permit heavy use.

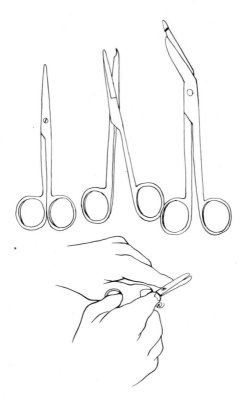

Silk sutures may be cut on the knot, but absorbable sutures require a tail to prevent unraveling. The scissors are opened slightly, the taut suture encountered, and the scissors run down until the knot is reached. The scissors are then twisted to raise the edge off the knot, and the suture material is divided.

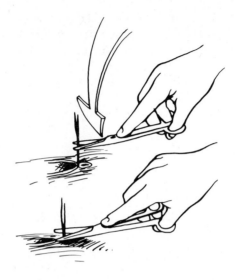

NEEDLE HOLDERS

Needle holders vary in size, depending on the tissue to be sewed and the depth of the incision. The needle holder is usually grasped with the thumb and fourth fingers through the rings, the third finger is placed outside one of the rings, and the index finger steadies the instrument. Control may require use of both hands when fine, delicate structures are sewed. Occasionally, the needle holder may be used in a palmed position that does not require placement of the fingers through the rings. This technique is more difficult to master. Curved needles should be passed with a twisting motion of the hand and wrist.

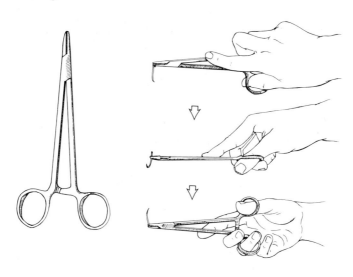

RETRACTORS

Retraction of most superficial structures can be effected with the use of three instruments. An Army-Navy retractor has two smooth, blunted ends angulated at 90° that vary in size to accommodate different structures. A vein retractor has a smooth but sharply curved tip that can retract cordlike structures. A rake retractor has teeth that may be either blunt or sharp and is most commonly used on skin. Operative circumstances dictate the type of retractor needed. Malleable retractors can be bent into different shapes.

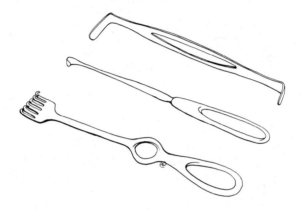

SUCTION TIPS

A tonsil suction has a blunt, multiply perforated end that is connected by a long neck to the handle. This instrument is commonly used to remove blood and other fluids from deep within a wound. A brain sucker, which has a vent on the side to control the amount of suction, is used for superficial work. Delicate suctioning can be accomplished with this instrument. A pencil sucker has a blunt tip connected to a straight tube and is used during suctioning of less delicate structures. It is held as a pencil.

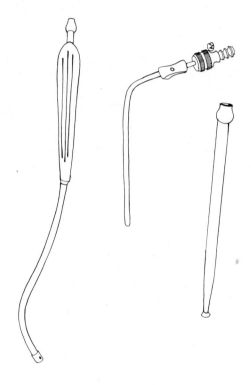

Suture Material

Suture material is of two types: absorbable and nonabsorbable. Catgut is the most frequently used absorbable suture. However, synthetic absorbable material that varies in reactivity and absorption has recently become available. Plain catgut is absorbed more quickly than chromic catgut, which is specially treated to retard absorption. Quickly absorbed material invokes a more intense inflammatory reaction than that absorbed slowly. In an infected field, absorbable sutures should be used; otherwise, nonabsorbable sutures will continue to be extruded, preventing wound healing, until they are all removed.

Suture material is available as loose strands or joined to needles. Nonabsorbable sutures include silk, cotton, wire, and synthetic filaments such as nylon. In the emergency department, silk and nylon are used for most skin closures. Knots may be securely placed with two or three throws of a silk suture; five or six loops are required to prevent unraveling of plastic sutures. When compared with catgut, silk sutures are relatively nonreactive; plastic sutures are less reactive than silk; and steel sutures are least reactive of all.

Commonly used sutures vary in diameter from 1-0 to 6-0, the smallest. Selection of the proper suture material depends on the tissue being handled:

Tissue	Size	Material
Deep fascia	1-0 or 2-0	Silk or chromic catgut
Superficial fascia	3-0	Silk or chromic catgut
Subcutaneous ties	3-0 or 4-0	Silk or plain catgut
Subcuticular skin closure	3-0 or 4-0	Plastic or plain catgut
Skin		
Scalp	2-0 or 3-0	Silk
Face	5-0 or 6-0	Silk or plastic
Back	2-0 or 3-0	Silk
Torso	3-0 or 4-0	Silk
Extremities	4-0 or 5-0	Silk or plastic

Needles

Needles are grouped according to size, shape, and type of point. Straight needles with cutting-edge tips are used for approximating skin edges. The long, straight needle can be easily grasped with the fingers and does not require the use of a needle holder. Curved needles may also be used to suture skin and are always employed when suturing deeper structures. A needle holder is required when using this type of needle.

Needles with cutting-edge tips are more easily passed through skin and other firm structures than are those without such tips. However, the cutting edge can lacerate blood vessels. Tapered, round-tipped needles are used for suturing fasciae and subcutaneous tissue. When passed through tissue, they push the blood vessels aside, avoiding injury and hemorrhage.

The curved, round tapered point is used for suturing subcutaneous tissue and fasciae; a curved or straight needle with a cutting-edge tip is used to suture skin.

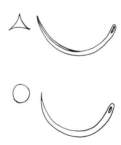

Suture material may be attached to the needle in three different ways: (1) The suture may be threaded through the eye; this requires a steady hand. (2) A French-eye needle has a slit end that is corrugated in such a manner as to permit a large thread to be looped onto it and be held securely in position. (3) A swaged-on needle has the thread already attached to the end, so that there is no double thread to be pulled through tissue. This type of needle-and-thread combination is less traumatic to tissue than the other types.

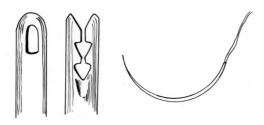

Knots

Two-hand knots, one hand knots, and knots tied with an instrument are the basic types of knots. Slip knots, surgeon's knots, and other types are not required for most emergency department procedures. Silk may be securely tied with a single square knot; absorbable suture material may require three or four knots. Plastic sutures often require five to seven knots if one is to be sure that the tie will not unravel. When tying individual sutures, silk is the easiest and fastest suture material to use, since it handles so well. A running suture is, of course, the fastest method of wound closure and can provide accurate skin approximation if performed properly.

TWO-HAND SQUARE KNOT

The two-hand square knot is preferred by most surgeons for tying a secure knot under excellent control. The strands are uncrossed, and each is held in a separate hand between the index finger and thumb.

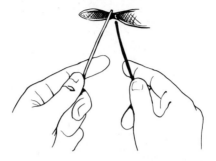

The right strand is looped under the left index finger and the right hand moves to the left.

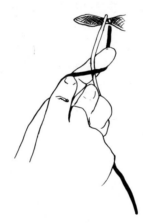

The left index finger and thumb are joined.

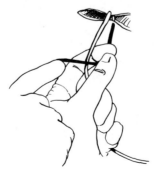

The thumb and index finger are passed back through the loop, and the right hand moves once again back to the right.

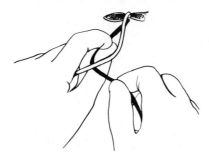

The right hand moves forward to place its strand between the pinched thumb and index finger of the left hand.

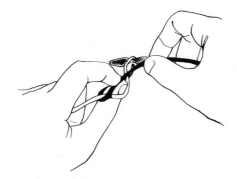

The right hand releases its strand, and this strand is then brought through the loop by the pinched index finger and thumb of the left hand and grasped once again by the right hand. The right-hand strand is then crossed over the left-hand strand.

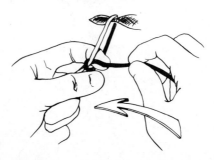

The knot is laid down. It is impossible to place a square knot without crossing the hand at some point during placement of the knot. If the hands never cross, a square knot is impossible.

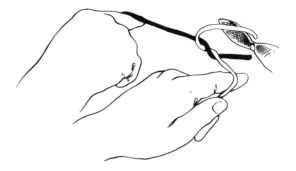

The left-hand strand is looped under the left thumb, and the right-hand strand is brought across the top surface of the left thumb by moving the right hand to the right.

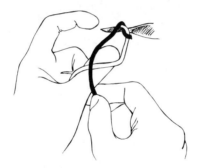

The thumb and index finger of the left hand are pinched.

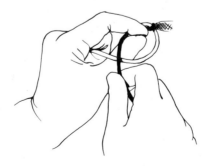

The two fingers are then brought through the loop, after which the right strand is placed between the pinched index finger and thumb of the left hand.

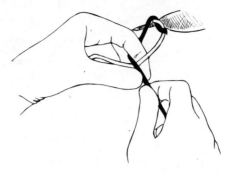

The right hand releases its strand, which is then brought through the loop between the index finger and thumb of the left hand.

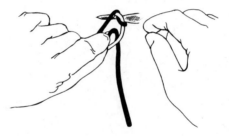

The right hand picks up its strand, and the knot is laid down with the left hand moving to the left and the right hand to the right. The square knot is completed.

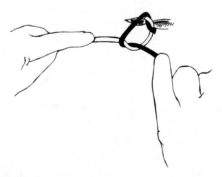

ONE-SQUARE KNOT

A one-hand square knot is faster to tie than a two-hand knot. The two strands are grasped with the left strand placed between the thumb and index fingers of the left hand and the right strand placed between the thumb and index finger of the right hand. The right strand lies over the third and fourth fingers.

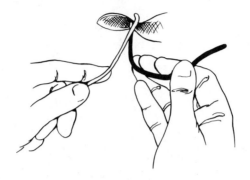

The left strand is placed across the surface of the third finger of the right hand, and the tip of the third finger is then flexed.

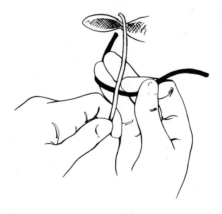

The right-hand strand is then looped onto the back of the distal phalanyx of the third finger by moving the thumb and index finger forward and then back again.

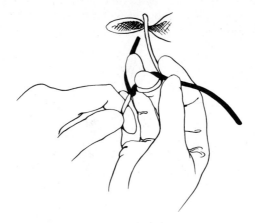

The knot is laid down by moving the left hand down and to the left and the right hand up and to the right.

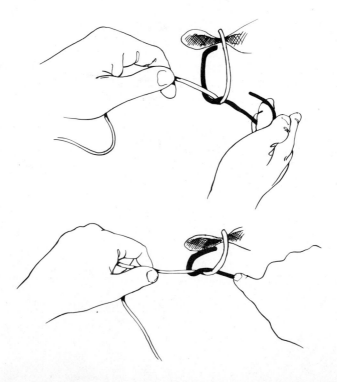

The right-hand strand is looped over the top of the index finger.

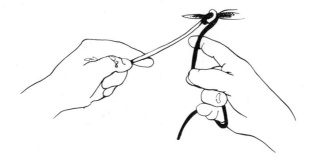

The right index finger is then flexed.

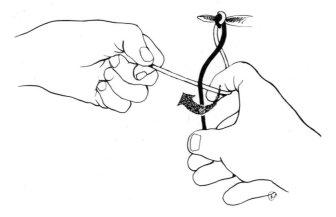

With the left-hand strand looping over the top of the right index finger, the right-hand strand is brought under the tip of the index finger, and the tip is then extended, causing the right strand to be brought through the loop.

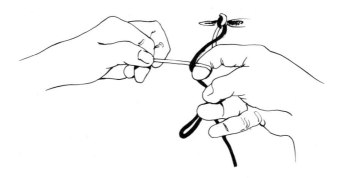

The right-hand strand is grasped between the index and third fingers and traction applied.

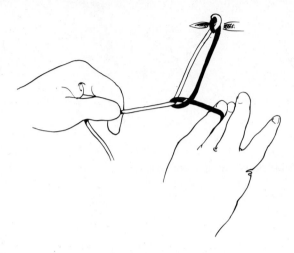

The left hand crosses over the top of the right hand to secure the square knot.

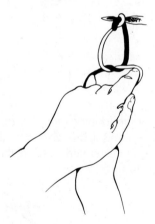

INSTRUMENT KNOT

The needle holder is held in the right hand, and a loop is started around the needle with the left-hand strand.

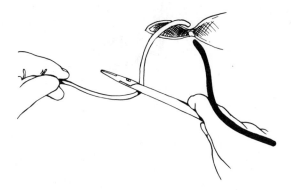

The loop around the end of the needle holder is completed.

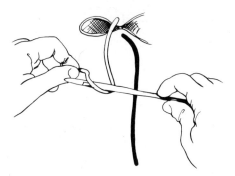

With the loop held in place, the right strand is grasped with the needle holder.

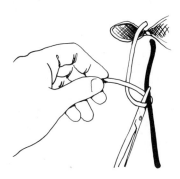

The right strand is then brought through the loop, and the needle holder passes above and to the left while the left hand crosses over the right and passes downward and toward the right.

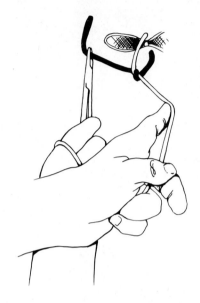

The loop is tightened.

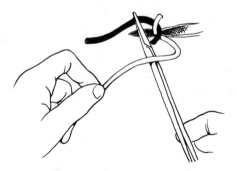

The right strand is released from the tip of the needle holder, and the left strand is looped around the needle holder. The right strand is picked up again with the needle holder.

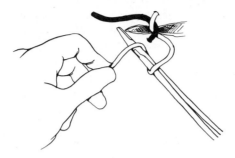

The right strand is then pulled through the loop, and the square knot is completed by tightening with the left hand and the needle holder.

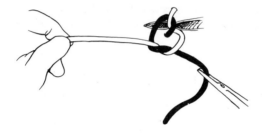

Wound Care

A complete examination of the patient, including an accurate history of allergic reactions to local anesthetics, is essential. Replacement of blood loss, intravenous fluid administration, and general medical care are important but beyond the scope of this discussion. Proper attire with a surgical cap, a mask, and sterile gloves is mandatory. Clean wounds are basically those treated within 8 hours, are not unduly contaminated, and do not involve farm injuries or animal bites. They can be closed primarily. Wounds that are older than 12 hours, result from animal bites, occur on farms, or involve massive tissue destruction, often require cleaning, debridement, and secondary closure, which should be supervised by a specialist. Although the number of different types and locations of wounds from trauma and surgical procedures are numerous, certain basic surgical principles apply to all situations. To emphasize these principles, the treatment of an arm laceration is reviewed.

The initial treatment is always to control hemorrhage. Direct pressure applied to the laceration is effective in almost all circumstances.

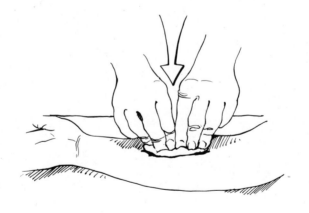

A tourniquet is almost never required to stop bleeding, and if applied tightly enough to stop it, impairs all blood flow to the extremity. Equally deleterious is a tourniquet with insufficient pressure that permits arterial inflow yet causes venous hypertension, thus resulting in increased hemorrhage.

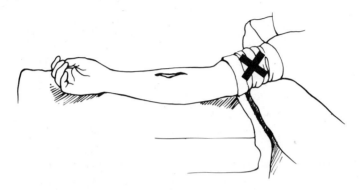

Careful inspection of the extremity, both in the area of the wound as well as distally, is essential. Palpation of the radial and ulnar arteries in the wrist will identify blood flow in this area. However, the presence of a pulse does not eliminate a possible proximal arterial injury. Arterial communicating arches in the wrist and palm permit enough collateral flow to result in pulsations of either artery should the opposite artery be ligated or injured. In the Allen test, both the radial and ulnar arteries are compressed while the patient's hand is opened and closed, thus draining it of blood. When one vessel is released, the hand should fill with blood immediately; failure to do so indicates that the hand depends on blood flow through the obstructed artery, and ligation of this vessel would be dangerous. In most circumstances, however, the radial or ulnar artery can be ligated without complications (see Chap. 3).

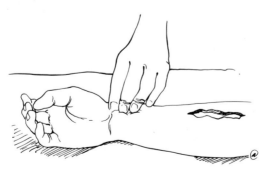

Testing movements of the patient's hand and fingers including the ability to oppose the thumb to the other fingers will identify potential tendon or motor nerve injury. Ability to perform gross and fine movements of the fingers indicates the absence of any significant injury to the tendons or to the intrinsic motor innervation of the hand.

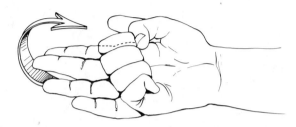

The hand is tested with a pin to determine if there is any sensory loss due to median, ulnar, or radial nerve injury. This must be completed before the wound is anesthetized to avoid inaccurate findings. If there is evidence of vascular, tendon, or nerve damage, further surgical consultation should be obtained. Otherwise, the wound may be prepared for cleaning, debridement, and closure. Heavily contaminated wounds, particularly those incurred during farm injuries, are often cleaned, debrided, and left open because of the high incidence of infection when primary closure is attempted.

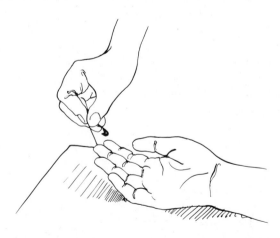

After obtaining hemostasis, the skin around the laceration is shaved, with care taken to keep hair from entering the wound.

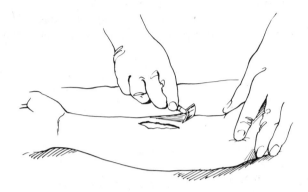

The sterile setup that is used contains soap and water for cleaning the wound, sterile saline for irrigation, basins, and irrigating syringes.

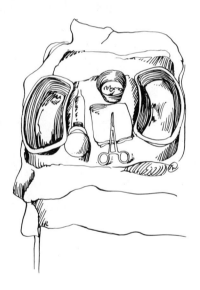

The area around the wound is scrubbed with soap and water to remove any grease, dirt, or other foreign material. If soap and water enter the wound, they are later washed away. If the wound is exquisitely painful, preliminary infiltration of a local anesthetic may be necessary before proper cleaning can be completed.

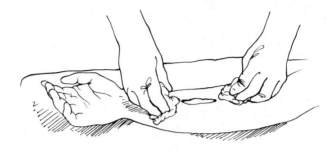

The wound is thoroughly irrigated with copious amounts of sterile saline to remove foreign material and to dilute the bacterial concentration. At this time, the dislodgment of clots may result in recurrent hemorrhage.

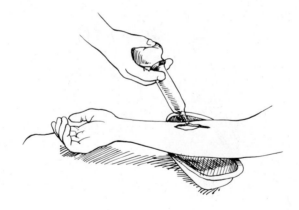

The basic surgical setup for debridement and closure of a laceration consists of an eye sheet to drape the area, sponges, cotton balls, antiseptic solution, assorted hemostats, an irrigating syringe, tissue forceps, dissecting scissors, suture scissors, a needle holder, scalpel handle and blade, suture material, syringes, needles, and an injectable local anesthetic.

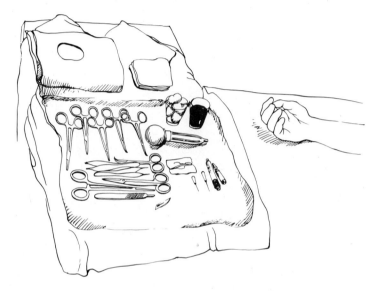

An antiseptic solution is applied around the wound to sterilize the field. Application of the antiseptic solution into the wound itself is best avoided, since it may result in damage to exposed tissue. A wide operative area should be prepared, since there is no disadvantage in preparing too large an area, but a distinct disadvantage in preparing one that is too small, particularly when it later proves necessary to enlarge the operative site.

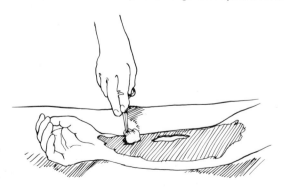

After preparation and draping, the wound is infiltrated with local anesthesia. Lidocaine, 0.5 or 1.0%, is commonly used. Epinephrine (1:100,000) is only infrequently added and should never be used in the penis or digits. Each side is injected through the skin or open wound. The injected local anesthetic easily diffuses through the tissues, and one or two needle sticks, rather than multiple punctures, usually suffice.

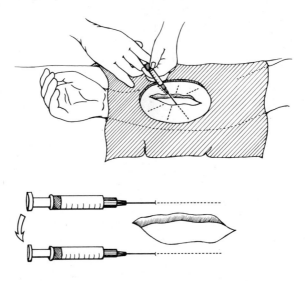

The wound is debrided, hemostasis obtained, and the wound closed by approximating first the deep structures and then the skin.

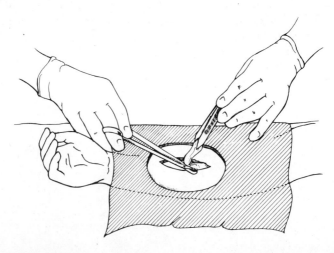

A dry sterile dressing is applied. The wound should be examined in 48 hours to ensure that proper healing is taking place and that there is no infection.

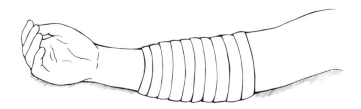

Wound Closure

A few basic techniques for deep tissue and skin approximation will enable most wounds to be closed without difficulty. Selection of appropriate suture material and needles has been outlined previously. Whether the wound is the result of trauma or an operation, it is essential to approximate only viable tissues and to eliminate dead space.

Ragged, irregular wounds are debrided back to bleeding tissue. A knife blade, not a scissors, should be used for this dissection to avoid skin-edge trauma (A). Hemostasis is secured with vascular clamps (B), and the vessels are ligated with fine silk or absorbable suture material (C). The wound is now ready for approximation of the subcutaneous tissue and skin.

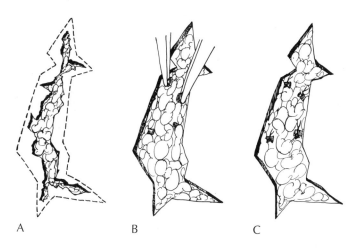

A   B   C

The epidermis, dermis, subcutaneous fat, and fascia are distinct layers that require accurate approximation (A). The thickness of the layers will vary according to the area of the body. The fascia is approximated first with interrupted, usually absorbable, suture material (B). The fatty subcutaneous layer is also joined with interrupted absorbable suture material (C). Finally, the epidermis and dermis are approximated by sutures placed through the skin (D).

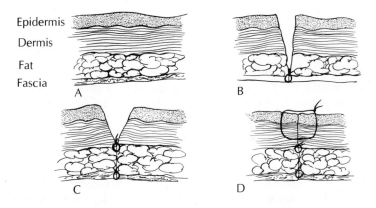

Epidermis

Dermis

Fat

Fascia

A   B

C   D

Wounds of significant length are closed by placing sutures at spaced intervals to divide the wound equally (A). Additional sutures are then inserted to approximate the skin edges accurately (B). Closing a wound continuously from one end to the other may result in inaccurate approximation of the edges if spacing sutures are not used.

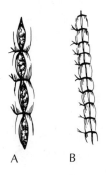

A   B

The most frequently used skin-closure techniques include the following: interrupted sutures (A); a running continuous suture (B); interrupted vertical mattress sutures in which one bite is taken away from the skin edge and the other at the skin edge (C); interrupted horizontal mattress sutures (D); a subcuticular closure in which a running suture is placed by taking bites of the dermis (E); and a continuous locking suture (F). As a rule, interrupted vertical mattress sutures have proved most effective in accurate skin edge approximation with minimal tension and distortion.

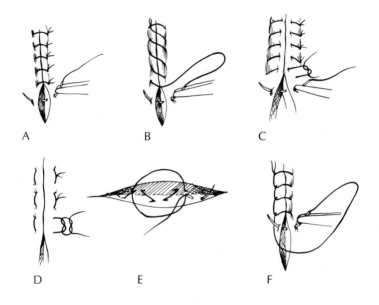

A   B   C

D   E   F

Instrument ties will greatly facilitate skin closure, especially when an assistant is not available. Accurate placement and tightening of the suture until there is appropriate tension is important. However, excessively tight wound closures will result in edema and strangulation of tissue.

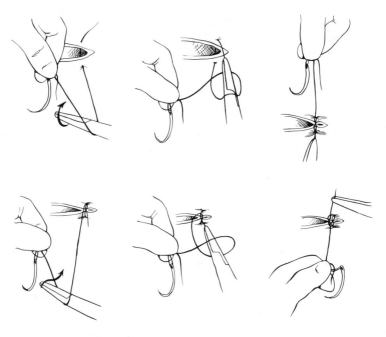

Certain general rules for suture removal can be applied. In face and neck wounds, every other suture is removed on day 2 or 3, and the remainder on day 4 or 5, to reduce the chance of crosshatch scarring. On the torso, sutures are left in place for 7 to 10 days and in the extremities, for 10 to 14 days, with the longer interval applying to more peripherally located wounds.

5

Regional Anesthesia

Richard A. E. Assaf

The two drugs most frequently employed to provide local analgesia are lidocaine and mepivacaine. Vasoconstricting agents, such as epinephrine, may be added to these local analgesic solutions to delay their absorption and also to prolong their action. This must *not* be done for regional blocks of the fingers or toes. Detoxification occurs in the liver and liver disease may increase the toxicity of these drugs. The blocking quality of a local analgesic drug will depend on its potency, latency (the time between its injection and minimal effect), and duration of action.

Precautions in the Use of Local Anesthetic Drugs

Local anesthetic techniques require the same sterile precautions as those for the operation. Aspiration is essential before all injections. Accidental rapid intravascular injection might be sufficient to produce a severe toxic reaction. Do not give more than the stated dose (in milligrams per kilogram of body weight). Once the local compound has been administered, the patient must not be left unattended.

Resistance to injection, combined with paresthesia, is likely to be due to an intraneural injection. When paresthesia has been elicited, the needle must be withdrawn a millimeter or two prior to injection to avoid disruption of nerve fibers.

Before any large volume of local analgesic solution is injected, the following should be available:

1. An open vein and fluid for infusion.
2. Tilting table or cart.
3. Facilities for the administration of oxygen by positive pressure and endotracheal intubation.
4. Suction equipment and catheters.
5. Syringes, needles, and drugs, such as amobarbital sodium (Amytal Sodium), succinylcholine (Anectine), diazepam (Valium), and vasopressors.

Complications of Local Anesthetics

All local analgesic drugs are, to a greater or lesser extent, toxic substances. The major cause of systemic reactions to these local compounds is a high blood concentration of the drug. This is more common after topical analgesia of the upper air passages and trachea than after local infiltration or nerve block. This is because absorption from the bronchial tree is almost as rapid as from intravenous injection. Signs of toxicity due to special sensitivity of the patient to the drug are rarely observed.

FACTORS INFLUENCING TOXICITY
Toxic signs may not always be related to dosage. The following factors influence toxicity:

1. Quantity of the solution
2. Concentration of the drug.
3. Presence or absence of epinephrine.
4. Vascularity at the site of injection.
5. Rate of absorption of the drug.
6. Rate of destruction of the drug.
7. Hypersensitivity of the patient.
8. Age, physical status, and weight of the patient.

Convulsions and cardiovascular and respiratory collapse are the most serious complications.

TREATMENT OF SYSTEMIC REACTIONS
Central Nervous System
Central nervous system toxicity is followed by depression, restlessness, hysterical behavior, vertigo, tremor, convulsions, and respiratory failure. Treatment consists of (1) artificial ventilation with oxygen and (2) sufficient amobarbital sodium to control convulsions (0.5 to 1 gm intravenously). Diazepam (5 to 10 mg intravenously) may be used instead of amobarbital sodium.

Cardiovascular System

The manifestations of acute collapse from primary cardiac failure include feeble pulse, bradycardia, pallor, sweating, and hypotension. This form of reaction may be caused by the rapid absorption of the drug, so that the cardiovascular system is involved before the drug has had time to reach the brain. Treatment consists of elevation of the legs, administration of oxygen, rapid intravenous infusion, use of a vasopressor drug, and cardiac massage.

Respiratory System

Respiratory depression, when it occurs, may proceed to apnea from medullary depression. Endotracheal intubation and ventilation must be rapidly instituted.

Allergic Phenomena

Allergic reactions are rare and may take the form of bronchospasm, urticaria, or angioneurotic edema. Treatment includes the administration of epinephrine, hydrocortisone, and oxygen. It is important to remember that reactions to the vasoconstrictor drug may occur, which may take the form of pallor, anxiety, palpitations, tachycardia, hypertension, and tachypnea.

Minimizing Reactions

1. Do not exceed recommended dosages.
2. Avoid intravenous administration by injecting with a moving needle.
3. Aspirate frequently.
4. Preservatives, such as phenol, chlorocresol, or sodium sulfite, should be avoided when a large volume of local analgesic solution is injected.

Pharmacology of Local Anesthetics

LIDOCAINE

Solutions of 0.25 to 0.5% for infiltrations and 1 to 2% for nerve blocks are available with and without epinephrine (1:100,000 to 1:200,000). Toxicity is not great, but cardiovascular and central nervous symptoms of overdose may occur. Metabolism of lidocaine can give rise to the formation of methemoglobin, the average peak concentration ensuing within 4 to 6 hours after injection; however, cyanosis is rare. The duration of effect of a 1% solution is approximately 60 minutes with epinephrine.

The suggested minimal safe dose of lidocaine for a 70-kg man is as follows: with epinephrine, 7 mg per kilogram; without epinephrine, 3 mg per kilogram. The following volumes are considered safe for administration:

Percent Concentration Used	Milliliters of Solution
With epinephrine	
0.5	100
1.0	50
2.0	25
Without epinephrine	
0.5	40
1.0	20
1.5	13
2.0	10

MEPIVACAINE

When administering mepivacaine (Carbocaine), a dose of 5 mg per kilogram of body weight should not be exceeded. The following are suggested safe volumes:

Percent Concentration Used	Milliliters of Solution
0.5	80
1.0	40
2.0	20

Brachial Plexus Block–Axillary Approach

INDICATIONS

The brachial plexus block–axillary approach is a useful technique for operations on the hand, forearm, and the distal part of the upper arm. Axillary block produces excellent anesthesia for the reduction of fractures. The area of anesthesia following an axillary brachial plexus block is demonstrated (A).

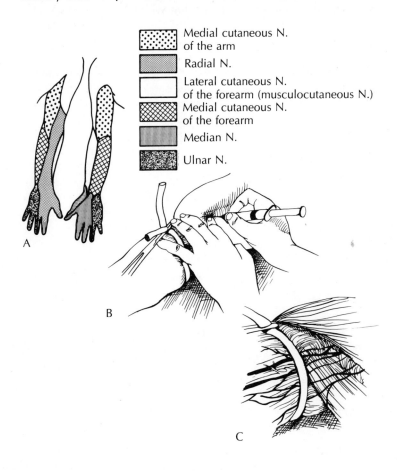

Medial cutaneous N. of the arm

Radial N.

Lateral cutaneous N. of the forearm (musculocutaneous N.)

Medial cutaneous N. of the forearm

Median N.

Ulnar N.

A

B

C

Only one landmark, the axillary artery, is used. No paresthesia is sought, so there is a reduced probability of nerve damage. Pneumothorax and phrenic nerve block does not occur. Pain is minimal during injection.

ANATOMY

In the axilla, the brachial plexus surrounds the axillary artery with three bundles, a medial, lateral, and a posterior bundle, from which the long nerves of the upper limb arise. The brachial plexus can be blocked between the axilla and the proximal part of the upper arm because the nerves lie in a relatively narrow fascial tube. The only exception is the musculocutaneous nerve carrying impulses to the radial side of the forearm, which leaves the plexus in the cephalad part of the axillary fossa.

TECHNIQUE

The patient is placed in the supine position with the arm abducted to a right angle. The humerus is externally rotated and the elbow flexed after the skin of the axilla has been cleaned and shaved. The axillary artery is palpated and a skin wheal raised at the highest part of the axilla at which the arterial pulsation is felt, proximal to the lower border of the pectoralis major. As the needle is inserted, the index finger of the opposite hand fixes the artery against the humerus. A short needle (2.5 to 5 cm) is then inserted toward and slightly above the artery either until a click is felt or marked pulsation of the needle is observed, which indicates that its point lies near the artery (B). The sensation of a click indicates that the needle tip lies in the neuromuscular compartment. Local analgesic solution with epinephrine is injected. Should paresthesia be encountered, the needle point is in the correct position. Injection is not attempted until the needle has been withdrawn slightly.

Prior to the injection of the local anesthetic solution, a tourniquet should be tightly placed on the arm approximately 7.5 cm below where the arterial pulsation is felt (C). This is done to prevent the distal spread of the local anesthetic solution and to force it upward, increasing the chances of producing a successful block of the musculocutaneous nerve. The tourniquet should remain in place at least 10 minutes to allow enough time for the local anesthetic to be fixed to nerve tissues. After a successful block, there should be complete analgesia below the elbow joint.

This technique does not render the shoulder joint insensitive and consequently cannot be used for manipulations of this joint. If a tourniquet is required, it will be necessary to perform a subcutaneous ring injection at the level of the initial skin wheal.

Occasionally, the musculocutaneous nerve (C6), which is the contribution of the lateral cord of the plexus, is given off higher than usual and consequently escapes the effect of the block. It can be dealt with by injecting 10 to 15 ml of 1% lidocaine solution into the subcutaneous tissues from a point 2.5 cm distal to the crease of the elbow joint in the cleft between the tendons of the biceps and the brachioradial muscle where it becomes the lateral cutaneous nerve of the foream.

Occasionally it may be necessary to anesthetize the ulnar nerve distribution. This is accomplished by locating the nerve where it runs in its groove behind the medial epicondyle. After palpation of the nerve with the patient's elbow flexed, 5 to 10 ml of 1% lidocaine is injected via a very fine needle proximal to the ulnar nerve sulcus (to avoid the risk of neuritis). Paresthesia may be elicited radiating down the ulnar side of the forearm and little finger.

COMPLICATIONS
Arterial or vein puncture may produce systemic toxic reactions. Arterial puncture, should it occur, may reduce the chances of a successful block, but is not a sign to discontinue the block. If it does occur, the needle point should be withdrawn slowly, usually less than 0.5 cm, until no blood is obtained by aspiration. Then the needle should still be located in the neuromuscular compartment, and the injection of the local anesthetic solution can be completed. Failure to locate the sheath may be due to pushing the needle too deeply, since the plexus at this point lies superficially. Temporary obliteration of a palpable radial pulse by compression of the axillary artery either by bleeding or excessive volume may occur in children.

ANESTHETIC AGENTS
Either lidocaine or mepivacaine (10 to 50 ml of a 1.0 to 1.5% solution with epinephrine 1:200,000) can be used for adults. It is important not to exceed the maximal dosage of 500 mg for lidocaine or 400 mg for mepivacaine. In children, a dose of 3 to 5 mg of the local anesthetic agent per pound of body weight should not be exceeded.

ONSET AND DURATION OF EFFECT

Induction time is longer with an axillary than with a supra-clavicular approach to a brachial plexus block because the local anesthetic must diffuse to all branches of the plexus. This may take 25 to 30 minutes in the adult and somewhat less time in children.

Operating analgesia lasts from 90 to 180 minutes. Epinephrine and stronger concentrations of solutions will prolong the effect.

Wrist Block

Partial or complete wrist block, with a tourniquet, is useful for surgery of the hand, especially if motor function is required during the operation. It should be noted that an Esmarch bandage is tolerated on the forearm only for short periods of time.

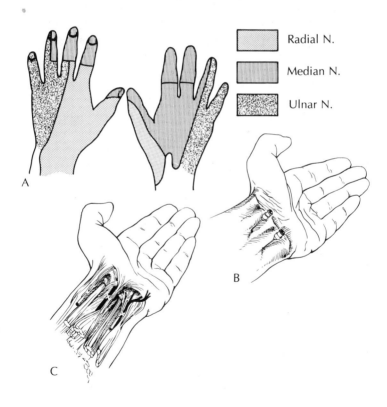

Radial N.

Median N.

Ulnar N.

A

B

C

MEDIAN NERVE

Anatomy

The median nerve at the level of the proximal crease comes to lie superficially on the anterior aspect of the wrist underneath or close to the radial side of the tendon of the palmaris longus. It lies medial to the tendon of the flexor carpi radialis muscle. The median nerve supplies the palmar surface of the fingers to the radial side of the midline of the ring finger, together with the skin over the dorsal aspects of the same fingers (A).

Technique

Identify the palmaris longus tendon by having the patient gently flex the wrist and simultaneously oppose the thumb. Direct a 25-gauge needle immediately to the radial side of the palmaris longus tendon at right angles to the skin and at the level of the proximal skin crease (B, C). Attempt to elicit paresthesia by moving the needle in a fanwise direction up and down in a plane at right angles to the long axis of the forearm. Inject 3 ml of 1% lidocaine, with or without epinephrine, even if paresthesia is not elicited.

ULNAR NERVE

Anatomy

In the forearm, about 5 cm above the wrist, the ulnar nerve divides into superficial terminal or palmar mixed and dorsal sensory branches. The palmar branch continues along the tendon of the flexor carpi ulnaris to divide on the radial side of the pisiform bone into a superficial and deep branch. The superficial branch, entirely sensory, is distributed to the ulnar side of the palmar aspect of the hand and to the palmar surfaces of the little finger and the ulnar side of the ring finger. The dorsal branch reaches the dorsal aspect of the wrist, supplying the ulnar side of the dorsum of the hand (A).

Technique

Gently flex the wrist and palpate the flexor carpi ulnaris. Insert a 25-gauge needle at right angles to the skin about 1 to 2 cm proximal to the wrist crease at the radial side of the tendon of the flexor carpi ulnaris and medial to the ulnar artery (B, C). If paresthesia is elicited, the needle should be redirected and 5 to 10 ml of 1% lidocaine injected. If no paresthesia is found, the same amount of solution can be injected while the point of the needle is drawn up from contact with the deep fascia and bone until it lies subcutaneously.

To block the dorsal branch of the ulnar nerve, a ring of local anesthesia, 5 ml of 0.5% lidocaine with or without epinephrine, is placed subcutaneously around the ulnar border of the distal forearm.

RADIAL NERVE
Anatomy
About 7 cm proximal to the wrist, the radial nerve comes to lie under the skin on the extensor aspect of the lower forearm and wrist. Here it breaks into several branches that supply the radial side of the dorsum of the hand, thumb, and index finger.

Technique
Inject 5 ml of 1% lidocaine with a vasoconstrictor between the skin and bone on the posterolateral aspect of the wrist joint near the base of the thumb lateral to the radial artery. The ring infiltration should not extend around the whole circumference of the wrist, and care should be taken not to injure subcutaneous veins. It is unwise to perform a wrist block in the presence of neuritis or carpal tunnel syndrome.

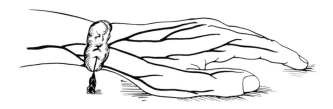

Digital Block

Anatomy

The digits are supplied by four nerve branches: two dorsal, which supply the back of the fingers, and two palmar, which supply the front. The dorsal nerves are terminal branches of the radial and ulnar nerves. The anterior nerves are terminal branches of the median and ulnar nerves. Epinephrine must not be used, since vasospasm and ischemia can occur.

Technique

Raise an intradermal wheal on the dorsum of the finger near its base with a 2-cm, 25-gauge needle. Inject 3 to 5 ml of 1 or 2% lidocaine through the wheal into the substance of the finger between bone and skin (A). Pass the needle downward until it is felt on the palmar skin, which is not pierced. After deposition of the solution, it may take up to 15 minutes for analgesia to be fully established.

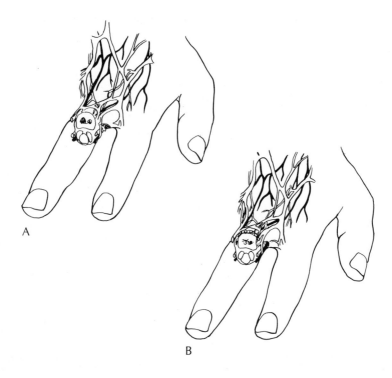

A

B

Another method of blocking the finger is to deposit 5 to 7 ml of a 1% lidocaine solution in each side of the interosseous space, entering from the dorsal aspect and carrying the needle almost to the palmar skin (B). Spread of infection due to this technique is very rare, provided that the solution is not injected into infected tissue.

If a tourniquet is used, no more than 3 ml of solution should be injected; a tourniquet must not remain on the finger for more than 15 minutes. It should not be used at all in patients with Raynaud's disease.

A similar technique using less solution can be employed on the toe.

Ankle Block

The nerves supplying the foot region can be blocked with relative ease at the ankle. This type of block is suitable for operations on the foot.

TIBIAL NERVE
Anatomy
The tibial nerve reaches the distal part of the leg after crossing under the Achilles tendon. Here it lies behind the posterior tibial artery, between the tendons of the flexor digitorum longus and flexor hallucis longus muscles, covered by the laciniate ligament. The medial calcaneal branch to the inside of the heel is given off at this point. The nerve then divides at the back of the medial malleolus into the medial and lateral plantar nerves, both of which run down to supply the side of the foot (A).

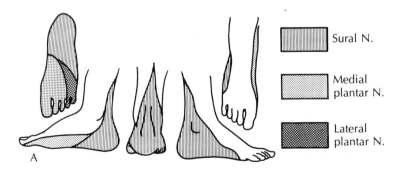

Sural N.

Medial plantar N.

Lateral plantar N.

A

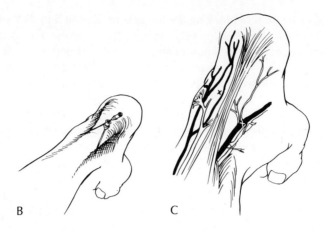

B   C

Technique
Place the patient in the prone position and attempt to palpate the
posterior tibial artery. Next, raise a skin wheal lateral to the
artery, or if the artery is not palpable, immediately to the lateral
side of the Achilles tendon at a level with the upper border of the
medial malleolus. Insert a fine-gauge needle, 6 to 8 cm long, at
right angles to the posterior aspect of the tibia, placing it immediately lateral to the posterior tibial artery (B). Attempt to elicit
paresthesia by moving the needle in a mediolateral direction.
When this is found, inject 5 to 10 ml of 0.5 or 1% lidocaine. If no
paresthesia is encountered, deposit 10 to 15 ml of the solution
against the posterior aspect of the tibia while the needle is drawn
back 1 cm.

Onset of anesthesia occurs between 10 and 30 minutes, depending on whether or not paresthesia was found. The area of anesthesia comprises mainly the sole of the foot, except for its most
proximal and lateral parts.

SURAL NERVE
Anatomy
The sural nerve supplies an area of skin along the outer margin of
the foot.

Technique
The nerve can be blocked by means of a subcutaneous infiltration stretching from the Achilles tendon to the outer border of the
lateral malleolus (B, C). Inject 8 to 10 ml of 0.5 or 1.0% lidocaine

with epinephrine via a fine-gauge needle while moving it in a fanwise fashion within the subcutaneous tissue between the lateral malleolus and Achilles tendon.

DEEP PERONEAL NERVE
Anatomy
The deep peroneal nerve innervates the short extensors of the toes, as well as the skin on the lateral side of the big toe and on the medial side of the second digit.

Technique
The deep peroneal nerve is blocked by inserting a 5-cm, 22-gauge needle midway between the most prominent points of the medial and lateral malleoli while directing it medially toward the anterior border of the medial malleolus (B). Deposit 10 to 15 ml of 0.5% lidocaine with epinephrine between the bone and skin. Paresthesia may or may not be elicited as the position of the nerve is not constant.

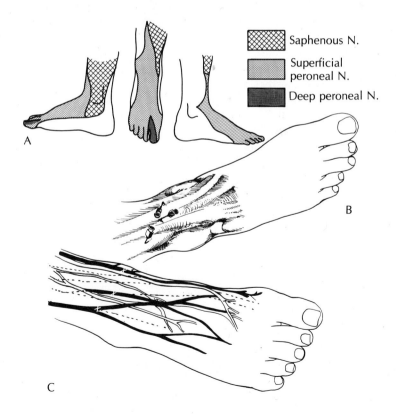

⬚⬚⬚ Saphenous N.

▓▓▓ Superficial peroneal N.

▓▓▓ Deep peroneal N.

SUPERFICIAL PERONEAL NERVE
Anatomy
The superficial peroneal nerve supplies the entire dorsum of the foot except for the small area of the skin that is innervated by the deep peroneal nerve (A).

Technique
The nerve is blocked by the subcutaneous infiltration of 5 to 10 ml of 0.5 or 1.0% lidocaine, extending from the anterior border of the tibia to the lateral malleolus (B, C).

SAPHENOUS NERVE
Anatomy
The saphenous nerve supplies an area of skin just above and below the medial malleolus (A).

Technique
Infiltrate subcutaneously 5 to 10 ml of 0.5 or 1.0% lidocaine around the great saphenous vein immediately above the medial malleolus (B, C). There is a risk of accidental intravenous injection; therefore, aspiration is essential.

Infiltration Anesthesia
Infiltration anesthesia is an ideal method for most minor surgical operations such as excision of small tumors and suturing of wounds. It requires injection of a local anesthetic and solutions into the cutaneous and subcutaneous tissues.

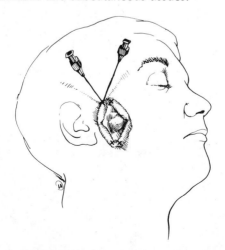

TECHNIQUE
To induce anesthesia for the removal of minor defects in the skin, such as cutaneous or subcutaneous tumors, the drug is infiltrated fanwise from two points, one above and one below the lesion.

DOSAGE
Dilute solutions of lidocaine (0.25 or 0.5%) with a vasoconstrictor are used for infiltration anesthesia. Again, it is imperative not to exceed the maximal dose. Also, necrosis of the wound edge has been observed following the injection of very large volumes of lidocaine with epinephrine. Therefore, the epinephrine concentration should not exceed 1:200,000. *For minor excisions and incisions,* 5 ml of 1.5% lidocaine or 30 ml of 0.25% lidocaine with epinephrine, 1:200,000, should be used. For *more extensive excisions,* 30 to 200 ml of 0.25% lidocaine, or 30 to 100 ml of 0.5% lidocaine, both with epinephrine, 1:200,000, is recommended.

CONTRAINDICATIONS
There are no special contraindications. For tissues supplied by end arteries, i.e., the toes and fingers, a local anesthetic solution without a vasoconstrictor should be used.

ASPIRATION TESTS
It is important to attempt to aspirate blood prior to the injection of each bolus of local anesthetic. It is possible that aspiration may be strong enough to collapse the wall of the vessel against the bevel, so that blood is not obtained. However, where a field block or local injection is being executed and the needle and syringe are moving backward and forward constantly, aspiration is not important. It is highly unlikely that the needle point will remain in a blood vessel sufficiently long to allow the injection of a toxic amount of solution.

Intravenous Regional Anesthesia

INDICATIONS

Intravenous regional anesthesia is a simple technique for operations, particularly below the elbow joint and knee and on the foot. A particular advantage of this technique is that the rapid termination of anesthesia (5 to 10 minutes) after the cuff has been deflated makes it possible to assess nerve and tendon function immediately after the operation. It can also be used for the reduction of fractures, repair of tendons, and suturing of wounds.

CONTRAINDICATIONS

Intravenous regional anesthesia is unsuitable in patients with a known history of hypersensitivity to local anesthetic agents and in those suffering from peripheral vascular or neurologic disease. The local anesthetic solution must *not* contain epinephrine.

TECHNIQUE

A blood pressure cuff is applied to the limb proximal to the site of operation, an indwelling 16- or 18-gauge cannula is inserted into a peripheral vein, and the limb is elevated to decrease the blood content. If a bloodless field is required, this may be achieved by the use of an Esmarch bandage. If the limb is too painful, simple elevation with applied pressure on the brachial artery (upper limb) will allow sufficient drainage of blood. Following this, the blood pressure cuff is inflated to at least 50 mm Hg above the systolic pressure. The pressure required will depend on the muscle mass component. It is obvious that a larger muscle mass, such as in the leg, needs a higher pressure to occlude the arterial blood pressure than does a small muscle mass. An efficient tourniquet does not completely isolate the limb because of the collateral circulation through bone.

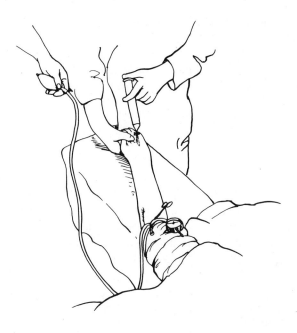

The local anesthetic solution can be given as a single dose through the cannula. It is perhaps wise in certain surgical procedures to leave the catheter in place and occlude it with a stopcock; this allows for the administration of supplementary doses if surgery is extended.

The pressure of the cuff usually becomes uncomfortable after 30 minutes. This discomfort may be eliminated by applying another cuff distal to the original one on an anesthetized portion of skin. A second method is to inject a circular band of local analgesic solution around the upper margin of the supplementary cuff.

DOSAGE

The quantity of solution given will depend on the volume of the limb. A suitable dose for the upper limb, when the cuff is applied around the middle part of the upper arm, is 2 to 3 mg per kilogram. This is equivalent to approximately 40 ml of a 0.5% solution of lidocaine or mepivacaine. For the lower limb with mid-thigh occlusion, a dose of 5 to 6 mg per kilogram (50 to 60 ml) may be required.

In normal adults, operations on the fingers will require 50 to 60 ml. When the tourniquet is placed on the forearm or calf 30 and 50 ml of solution respectively should be sufficient. The more efficient the drainage of blood from the limb, the less the amount of local analgesic solution that will be required.

COMPLICATIONS
The risk of toxic reactions due to the sudden release of local analgesic solution into the circulation is ever present when the cuff is deflated. It is important to observe the patient carefully during and after the release of the cuff. The intermittent release of the tourniquet at 5-second intervals allows divided doses of the drug to be released and will increase the margin of safety. Treatment for toxic reactions has already been described. The signs of toxicity on releasing the tourniquet may include drowsiness, bradychardia, hypotension, and electrocardiograph abnormalities.

After the release of the cuff, peak levels are inversely proportional to the tourniquet time and tend to be lower with the 0.5% solution than with the 1.0% solution. The release of lidocaine is biphasic, consisting of an initial fast release of approximately 30 percent, followed by a gradual washout of the remainder. Even 30 minutes after the cuff is released, 50 percent of the dose may remain in the arm. Should it be necessary to reestablish anesthesia within 30 minutes of cuff release, this may be possible using half the initial dose.

Intercostal Nerve Block
Intercostal nerve block may be beneficial for patients suffering from painful fractured ribs, which hinder the respiratory effort.

ANATOMY
Each intercostal nerve is formed by the union of the anterior (motor) and posterior (sensory) roots. This mixed spinal nerve soon divides into anterior and posterior primary divisions.

In the thoracic region, the anterior branches of the second to sixth intercostal nerves run segmentally under the respective ribs, having crossed the paravertebral spaces between the necks of the contiguous ribs. At the anterior axillary line, each intercostal nerve gives off a lateral cutaneous branch and, at the end of the sternum, an anterior cutaneous one, as well as muscular branches to the intercostal muscles. The seventh to eleventh nerves pass below and behind the costal cartilages, between the internal oblique and transverse muscles, to enter the posterior layer of the rectus sheath. They run deep to the rectus muscle, pierce and supply it, and end as the anterior cutaneous nerves.

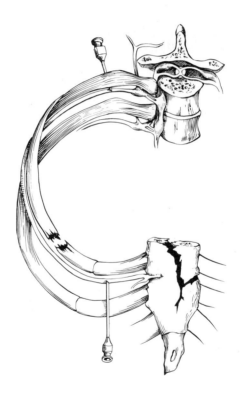

The lateral cutaneous nerves emerge in the midaxillary line, where they divide into anterior and posterior branches that supply the skin area of the lateral chest wall as far as the nipple line. The anterior cutaneous branches, which are the terminations of the intercostal nerves, supply the skin in front of the chest medial to the nipple line. The first thoracic nerve sends most of its fibers to the brachial plexus and has neither lateral nor anterior cutaneous branches. The skin supply over the first intercostal space is from the descending branches of the cervical plexus (C3 to C4). The lateral cutaneous branch of the second intercostal nerve becomes the intercostal brachial nerve after crossing the axilla.

TECHNIQUE

The intercostal nerves can best be blocked in the areas of the costal angles immediately lateral to the outer border of the sacrospinalis muscle. The patient may be placed on the side or in the prone position. However, this may be too painful a position for patients who have bilateral rib fractures. In such patients, the sitting position with a pillow held across the abdomen of the patient is most comfortable. An assistant may help support the patient's shoulders.

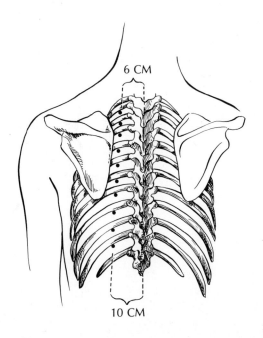

6 CM

10 CM

The patient's arm is drawn upward and forward to bring the scapula away from the region of the costal angles, so that it may be possible to block as far up as the fourth or fifth intercostal nerve. The lower margin of the ribs are then palpated with the fingers of one hand, and the overlying skin is drawn up cephalad. An intradermal wheal is raised over the lower border of the rib (approximately 4 fingerbreadths from the midline).

A fine needle is introduced until contact is made with the lower border of the rib. It is then partially withdrawn and advanced until it slips past the lower border of the rib to a depth of about 3 mm; 5 ml of 1% lidocaine with epinephrine is then injected while the needle point is slightly advanced and withdrawn so as to surround the nerve with the analgesic solution. It is important to have perfect control of the needle. This can be accomplished by placing one hand on the back while holding the hub of the needle between the thumb and index finger. The needle should be mounted on a syringe so that no air will enter the pleural cavity should the pleura be punctured.

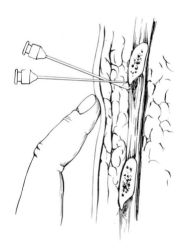

The twelfth spinal nerves are deeper and require special care.

COMPLICATIONS
The most important complication is pneumothorax, caused by lung puncture. An intercostal block must not be attempted if the rib cannot be felt with ease. It is important that the maximal dose for the local anesthetic not be exceeded.

6

Biopsies

Robert C. Wray, Jr.

Needle Biopsy

A sample from most of the solid visceral organs can be obtained by needle biopsy. However, needle biopsy is used most frequently for biopsy of the liver, bone marrow, prostate, kidney, parietal pleura, lung, breast, bone, and soft tissues. In general, needle biopsy has the following significant advantages over incisional or excisional biopsy: (1) shorter operative time; (2) performance under local anesthesia; (3) decreased likelihood of injury to associated structures; and (4) less cost to the patient. However, as with any invasive technique, significant hazards are associated with needle biopsy. These will be discussed subsequently.

Biopsies of the liver, kidney, pleura, and lung may be performed in the emergency department, but the patient must always be hospitalized for observation for 24 to 48 hours. These procedures usually require the attendance of a specialist.

GENERAL INDICATIONS AND CONTRAINDICATIONS

Detection of disease, most frequently malignant disease, is the usual indication for needle biopsy. Lack of patient cooperation is a relative contraindication to needle biopsy. Some patients tolerate the procedure without any premedication; others require extensive premedication, and some require general anesthesia. The patient should be questioned about bleeding during previous operations or tooth extractions and about bruising and bleeding from minor trauma and lacerations. Blood coagulation studies are not done before biopsy unless an abnormal history is obtained. Acute infection in the biopsy area is a relative contraindication to needle biopsy. Local infection can sometimes be circumvented by using a different route to perform the biopsy. Specific contraindications to the needle biopsy in a particular organ are given in the discussion of biopsy of that organ.

Technique

To perform a needle biopsy one needs equipment for cleaning the skin, drapes for the area of needle insertion, appropriate general or infiltration anesthesia, and the proper biopsy needle. The skin at the site of biopsy can be cleaned with hexachlorophene soap, Zephiran, Septisol, or Betadine scrub for 10 minutes. Sterile cloth towels or disposable towels or sheets are placed about the area of biopsy. Five different types of biopsy needles are generally used: long trephine (A), for lung and bone aspiration biopsy; Vim-Silverman (B) and Menghini (C), for needle biopsy of the liver; bone marrow, with long and short needles (D); and pleural biopsy (E). Disposable versions of many of these needles are now available.

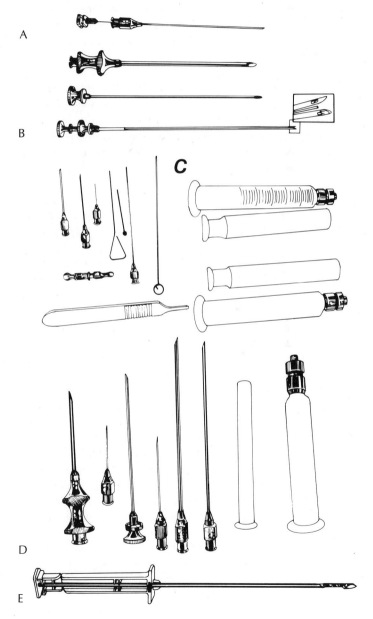

Complications

The most common complication of needle biopsy is inadvertent entry into some tissue other than the intended. Local bleeding and hematoma formation are also common. The most immediate and life-threatening complication is overdosage with, or an idiosyncratic reaction to, infiltration anesthesia. Organ system–specific complications are discussed in subsequent sections.

LIVER BIOPSY

Indications and Contraindications

Detection of cirrhosis or malignant disease is the most common indication for needle biopsy of the liver. Since liver function affects many of the factors involved in blood clotting, coagulation studies are usually obtained before liver biopsy. Liver biopsy should not be carried out in the presence of extrahepatic obstructive jaundice.

Technique

Liver biopsy can be performed either with the Vim-Silverman or Menghini needle; the latter is more frequently used. The patient is not allowed to eat or drink after midnight. The biopsy site is generally in the eighth or ninth intercostal space between the anterior and midaxillary lines. The area is prepared and draped. All tissues between the skin and the liver are infiltrated with local anesthesia.

If the Vim-Silverman needle (A) is used, the patient must be able to hold his breath for approximately 10 seconds. A small stab wound in the skin is made with No. 11 scalpel blade. With the obturator in place (B), the Vim-Silverman needle is introduced to just superficial to the liver (C), the obturator is removed (D), and the forked portion of the needle is inserted (E). The entire needle and forked portion are inserted into the liver for a distance of 2 to 3 cm (F). The forked portion of the needle is then advanced for an additional 1.5 cm while the outer barrel of the needle is held steady. Then the outer barrel of the needle is advanced over the forked needle in a rotating motion (G). The entire assembly is rotated 90° and withdrawn (H). A Band-Aid is applied, and the patient is observed for 24 hours.

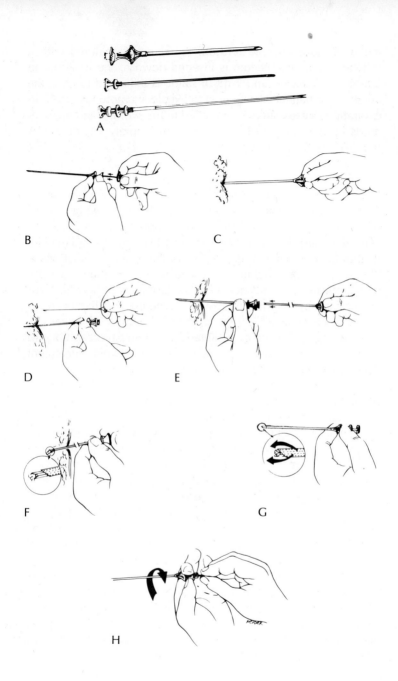

A

B

C

D

E

F

G

H

If the Menghini needle is used, the skin is punctured with a stylette, the biopsy needle is inserted down to the level of the intercostal muscles, and 1 ml of saline is infiltrated to clear the needle. The patient is instructed to exhale and hold his breath in expiration. Steady suction is applied to the syringe, and the needle is inserted quickly into the liver and rapidly withdrawn. A Band-Aid is then applied.

Complications

Hemorrhage is the most common fatal complication of liver biopsy. Hemorrhage occurs in approximately 0.1 to 0.2 percent of biopsies. Mortality from hemorrhage is approximately 0.03 percent. Bile leakage may occur following liver biopsy and may be fatal in approximately 0.02 percent of the patients. Other possible complications include hemorrhage into the pleural cavity, pneumothorax, and a "shocklike" syndrome. The shocklike syndrome may be a form of vasovagal syncope and has been reported to cause death. Rarely, puncture of other abdominal viscera, including the kidney, gallbladder, colon, pancreas, adrenal gland, lung, and small bowel, may occur. Very rarely is treatment needed for accidental puncture of other viscera.

BONE MARROW BIOPSY

Indications and Contraindications

Bone marrow biopsy is most often performed to diagnose diseases of the blood-forming system, including those involving the red blood cells (anemias, erythrocythemias), platelets (thrombocytopenia and thrombocytosis), and white blood cells (leukopenia and leukemias). The general contraindications apply.

Technique

Bone marrow biopsy is usually performed in the sternum or the iliac crest. With the patient in the supine position, the area is prepared and draped. A bone marrow biopsy needle is inserted through the outer table with gentle pressure. A definite decrease in resistance is felt as the marrow cavity is entered. The material is then aspirated using a syringe attached to the needle. Some material is immediately smeared; additional specimens may be fixed in formalin for examination by conventional techniques.

Complications

The posterior wall of the sternum can be transgressed and the heart or great vessels injured. Local bleeding is more common following biopsy of the iliac crest than of the sternum.

PROSTATE BIOPSY
Indications and Contraindications
The most common indication for prostate biopsy is the detection of prostatic carcinoma. The general contraindications apply.

Technique
The patient is generally placed in either the lithotomy or knee-chest position (Chap. 11). The biopsy can be done through the intact skin of the perineum, but is usually done transrectally. The technique of insertion of the Vim-Silverman needle is as shown for liver biopsy.

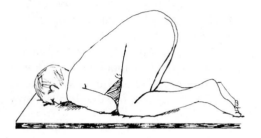

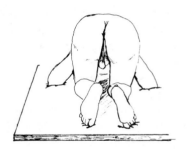

Complications
Bleeding is the most frequent complication, but is very rarely sufficient to dictate transfusion. All other complications are rare.

RENAL BIOPSY
Indications and Contraindications
Amyloidosis, glomerulonephritis, pyelonephritis, acute tubular necrosis, and the nephrotic syndrome can all be diagnosed by needle biopsy. Generally, needle biopsy should not be used to diagnose cancer of the kidney. Unilateral absence of a kidney and severe hypertension are relative contraindications to needle biopsy. Others are given under General Indications and Contraindications.

Technique
A preliminary exeretory urogram or plain x-ray film of the abdomen is necessary for the determination of the location of the kidneys. The patient is placed prone with a sandbag or folded sheet beneath the abdomen. This positioning brings the kidneys toward the back. The right kidney is usually chosen for biopsy because of the presence of other structures about the left kidney. Preparation and draping are routine. After adequate local anesthesia is obtained, the biopsy is obtained, usually with a Vim-Silverman needle.

Complications
The most common major complication is bleeding into the renal parenchyma or renal pelvis. Gross hematuria occurs in 5 to 10 percent of the patients, and the bleeding may obstruct the ureter or dictate transfusion. However, absolute bed rest and ingestion of large volumes of fluid will usually control the bleeding. In rare instances a nephrectomy has been required for severe bleeding. Deaths have also been reported to follow renal biopsy. Bacterial seeding with chills and fever is probably the most common complication.

PLEURAL BIOPSY
Indications and Contraindications
The most frequent indication is the need to diagnose infectious (primarily tuberculosis) or neoplastic disease involving the pulmonary system. The neoplastic disease may be diffuse or localized. Severe compromise of pulmonary function and other general contraindications to biopsy apply.

Technique

The patient is placed in the sitting position with the arms abducted to 90°, elbows flexed, and body leaning over a Mayo stand or bedside table. Routine preparation, draping, and infiltration anesthesia are used. The site of biopsy is dictated by abnormalities on the chest x-ray film. If no abnormalities of the pleura are visible, a biopsy specimen is taken just inferior to the tip of the scapula. The pleural biopsy needle is introduced first, then the sheath is retracted, and the hooked needle is pulled back to bite into the parietal pleura just superior to the rib, avoiding the neurovascular bundle. The sheath is then advanced in a manner similar to that used with the Vim-Silverman needle in liver biopsy and cuts off a portion of the pleura within the notch of the needle.

Complications

The most common complication is pneumothorax. Follow-up chest x-ray examination must be done after pleural biopsy. Hemothorax may occur secondary to laceration of an intercostal artery. Injury to the aorta or the vena cava is rare.

LUNG BIOPSY
Indications and Contraindications

The primary indication for lung biopsy is to determine the cause of diffuse lung disease. Biopsy of solitary pulmonary lesions may be done in patients who are not felt to be suitable candidates for thoracotomy. Severe limitation of pulmonary function and other general contraindications apply.

Technique

The procedure is done under sterile conditions and after adequate premedication and routine preparation and draping of the skin. Usually, lung biopsy is carried out under image-intensification fluoroscopy. Either the standard Vim-Silverman needle, using the technique previously described or a longer, Menghini needle can be used, applying continuous suction with an attached syringe.

Complications

Pneumothorax develops in approximately 25 percent of the patients. Follow-up chest x-ray studies must be done. Mortality of 0.5 to 1.0 percent has been reported.

BREAST BIOPSY
Indications and Contraindications
Almost all needle biopsies of the breast are done to confirm or rule out malignant disease. The usefulness of needle biopsy here is controversial. Many surgeons believe that incisional biopsy is indicated if a diagnosis of benign disease is obtained. However, if cancer is diagnosed, the need for incisional or excisional biopsy prior to mastectomy is obviated. The general contraindications to needle biopsy apply.

Needle breast biopsy should be distinguished from simple aspiration of breast masses. If the mass is aspirated and completely disappears, it can be assumed to be benign, and the patient can be examined again in a month.

Technique
Premedication is optional. The area is prepared and draped in routine sterile fashion. The Vim-Silverman needle biopsy technique is employed.

Complications
Rarely, a pneumothorax is produced by passing the needle through the breast mass and chest wall.

SOFT TISSUE MASSES
Indications and Contraindications
Various soft tissue masses, particularly lymph nodes and soft tissue tumors, can be examined by needle biopsy. The purpose is usually to determine whether or not the patient has malignant disease. Needle biopsy of soft tissue masses has not become popular. This lack of wide acceptance is probably a result of pathologists' difficulty in interpreting the material. Thus, most surgeons favor incisional or excisional biopsy.

Technique
The Vim-Silverman biopsy technique is used.

Complications
All complications are rare, but the most common is laceration of a vessel in the biopsy area and the formation of hematoma.

BONE

Indications and Contraindications

The primary indication for bone biopsy is to detect tumors that are metastatic to bone. Biopsy is occasionally performed to find the cause of diffuse bone disease. Rarely, the length of the needle may allow one to obtain tissue from a relatively inaccessible area, thus obviating the need for a major incisional biopsy. The general contraindications apply.

Technique

After premedication, preparation, and draping, the procedure can be carried out under local anesthesia for the thoracic and lumbar vertebrae. A long needle is inserted 6.5 cm from the midline on either side. The exploring needle is advanced 6 or 7 cm beginning at this point and inserted at a 125° angle from the horizontal. Anterior, posterior, and lateral x-ray films are then taken. If the needle is in the proper position, it is inserted 1.5 cm deeper while a partial vacuum is created in the biopsy needle syringe.

The technique for the upper thoracic vertebrae is similar, except that the needle is inserted 4 cm from the midline. Again, x-ray films are taken to determine the position of the needle.

Complications

Primary complications relate to entering either the kidney or one of the major abdominal vessels. Deaths have been reported following this procedure.

Incisional and Excisional Biopsy Techniques

Incisional (cutting into the lesion) or excisional (removing the entire lesion) biopsies can be used for any skin lesion and for selected lymph node, muscle, nerve, and arterial lesions. Usually, local anesthesia is sufficient, but regional or general anesthesia is sometimes used. Incisional techniques can be mastered by virtually any physician, but excisional techniques should only be performed by those with some experience in minor surgery.

INDICATIONS AND CONTRAINDICATIONS

Determination of the cause of disease is the most usual indication for incisional or excisional biopsy. As with needle biopsy, the most frequent indication is to determine whether or not the patient has malignant disease.

There are no absolute contraindications to this type of biopsy, but relative contraindications include acute infection in the region of the biopsy and a history of a severe bleeding disorder. Specific indications and contraindications are discussed under the tissues to be biopsied.

TECHNIQUE

Premedication is given, depending on the type of anesthesia, to be used. The skin is prepared and draped in the usual fashion. Incisional biopsies are virtually always taken with a scalpel, generally, with a No. 15 blade, but at times a No. 10, or No. 20 blade may be used. Occasionally, a skin punch can be used to remove a circular portion of skin. Other equipment required includes needle holders, fine hemostats (mosquito clamps), and tissue forceps (Adson forceps with multiple or 1 × 2 teeth).

COMPLICATIONS

The most common complication is development of a hematoma. The second most common is wound infection. Injury to any adjacent structure can occur.

SKIN BIOPSY

Indications and Contraindications

Most frequently, biopsies of skin lesions are done to determine whether or not the patient has a malignancy. Occasionally, biopsy specimens are taken for culture and for microscopic section to look for infectious or collagen disease. The general relative contraindications apply.

Technique

The majority of skin biopsies are excisional and performed for facial lesions. These biopsies generally should be made in the shape of a lenticular configuration (e.g., the cross section of a biconvex lens). The long dimension of the lenticular configuration is generally three times the short dimension. If possible, the long dimension should be oriented parallel to one of the wrinkle or crease lines of the face or neck.

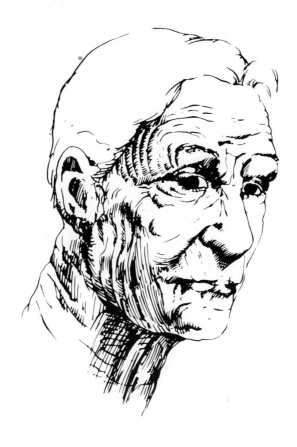

Premedication and routine preparation and draping are used. The area to be excised is outlined with a skin marking pencil or with methylene blue, brilliant green, or crystal violet. If a malignancy is suspected, a margin of 3 to 5 mm beyond the extreme limits of the gross disease should be removed. The depth of excision should allow removal of 1 to 2 mm of subcutaneous tissue.

Many techniques of wound closure are effective. Usually, subcuticular absorbable sutures of polyglycolic acid and simple skin sutures placed a millimeter apart and a millimeter back from the skin edges are sufficient. Sutures 4-0, 5-0, or 6-0 in diameter are used. Excision of lesions sufficiently large to make primary closure impossible is beyond the scope of this text.

Complications
Complications are rare, but wound infection and hematoma are the most common. Most uncommon are injuries to structures lying deep to the skin.

LYMPH NODE BIOPSY
Indications and Contraindications
Usually, lymph node biopsies are performed to establish the presence or absence of malignant disease. The second most common indication is to determine if the patient has an infectious disease (e.g., histoplasmosis, tuberculosis, cat-scratch fever). The general contraindications apply.

Technique
Lymph node biopsies are performed through a skin incision appropriate for the area of lymph node involvement. Generally, lymph nodes that are enlarged or suspected to contain a disease process are chosen for biopsy, although random lymph nodes

may sometimes be chosen. If the lymph node biopsy is to be done in the neck, the patient is placed on the operating table with the head turned to the side opposite the lesion.

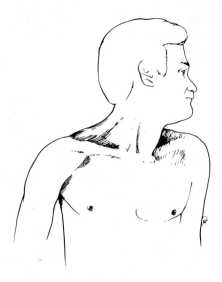

An incision parallel to the wrinkle line in the neck is generally chosen. Ideally, this incision should be placed so that it can be encompassed in a radical neck dissection incision later. If the lymph node biopsy is done in the axilla, the arm is abducted.

The incision can be placed either parallel or at right angles to the anterior axillary fold, but the latter is preferable.

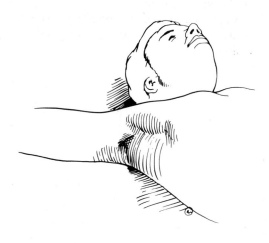

Inguinal lymph node biopsy is done with the patient supine and the incision made parallel to the inguinal ligament. Epitrochlear lymph node biopsy is performed on an abducted arm through an incision at right angles to the long axis of the arm. The incision is centered over the epitrochlear nodes (which generally lie approximately 4 cm proximal to the medial epicondyle).

After appropriate premedications and routine preparation and draping, the incision is made through the skin and subcutaneous tissues to expose the lymph node. In the inguinal, axillary, and epitrochlear areas there are usually no significant structures overlying the lymph nodes; in the neck the sternocleidomastoid muscle must occasionally be retracted. Blood vessels are clamped and either coagulated with electrocautery or ligated. Blood vessels that enter the hilus of the lymph node should be clamped and ligated before removing the node. The skin is closed as for an incisional biopsy of the skin.

Complications
Hematoma and wound infection are the most common complications. In the groin and epitrochlear areas, injury to underlying structures is unlikely. In the axillary area the axillary vein generally lies just deep to the lymph nodes and can be injured. In biopsy of the scalene lymph nodes in the neck, the transverse cervical artery can be divided causing hemorrhage or the dome of the pleura lacerated, resulting in a pneumothorax.

MUSCLE BIOPSY
Indications and Contraindications
Muscle biopsies are most frequently performed to determine the cause of muscular weakness or wasting. The general contraindications to an incisional biopsy apply.

Technique

A muscle that is believed to be involved by the disease process is usually chosen for biopsy. If a random biopsy is to be done, virtually any muscle may be used. However, a muscle that is covered by the thinnest amount of skin and subcutaneous tissue is usually selected. After adequate premedication and general, regional, or local anesthesia, routine preparation and draping are carried out. A skin incision is made and deepened through the subcutaneous tissue. Blood vessels are clamped and ligated or treated with electrocautery. An incision is made through the fascia of the muscle, and a segment of muscle, usually measuring approximately 3.0 × 0.5 cm, is removed. Removal of the muscle and fixation with its fibers under some tension usually make microscopic examination more precise. Tacking the stretched muscle to a piece of cardboard with four pins is a useful technique. Generally, the muscle fascia can be left unrepaired. If the defect is wider than 5 mm, repair with 4-0 polyglycolic acid suture is indicated. The skin and subcutaneous tissues are closed as previously outlined.

Complications

The most common complications are wound infection and hematoma. Rarely, a muscle fascia hernia may occur.

NERVE AND ARTERY BIOPSY

Indications and Contraindications

Nerve and artery biopsies are generally performed simultaneously. Microscopic examination of these tissues is used to determine whether or not the patient has collagen-vascular disease, polyneuritis, or other neurologic disorders. The general contraindications to incisional biopsy apply.

Technique

The sural nerve is most commonly chosen for biopsy, but any superficial cutaneous nerve (such as the lateral cutaneous nerve of the forearm) can be used. Appropriate premedication, anesthesia, and preparation and draping are completed. Two different incisions are made. If a simultaneous biopsy of the gastrocnemius muscle is not being done, an incision is made parallel to the course of the sural nerve just superior to the lateral malleolus. If gastrocnemius muscle biopsy is being performed, the incision is placed at the junction of the proximal and middle thirds of the leg and overlying the sural nerve. An incision 3 cm in length usually suffices for exposure of the nerve. Blood vessels are clamped and ligated or coagulated with electrocautery. A 2-cm portion of nerve is removed. A 1-cm segment of any blood vessel in the area can be removed for the vessel biopsy. If a muscle biopsy is being performed simultaneously, sufficient blood vessels are usually found in the muscle. The skin and subcutaneous tissues are closed in the usual technique.

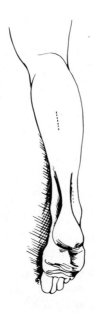

Complications

Not truly a complication but actually a sequela of removal of a cutaneous nerve is the development of an area of cutaneous hypoesthesia or anesthesia. If the sural nerve is removed, this usually involves the lateral aspect of the foot and the fourth and fifth toes. The area of distribution of the sural nerve is variable, and the area of numbness may be imperceptible or involve half the foot. If the lateral cutaneous nerve of the forearm is used, a small area of numbness develops on the distal forearm. The only other significant complications are wound infection and hematoma.

7

Nervous System Emergency Techniques

Allen P. Klippel

Analysis of the causes of death in highway accidents indicates that the leading cause is injury to the head followed closely by chest injuries. The proper handling of critically injured patients on the scene is mandatory if they are to arrive at the hospital alive. The emergency medical technician should have maintained a proper airway and administered oxygen during the transport interval. After the patient's arrival at the hospital, it is equally important to continue ventilation and stabilization of the patient's general condition before any diagnostic tests are performed. Blood for blood gas determinations and other indicated blood studies should be drawn before roentgenograms are made.

Classification of Central Nervous System Injuries

Injuries to the central nervous system are usually considered in three categories:

1. *Closed:* The scalp or mucous membranes are intact.
2. *Open:* The scalp or mucous membranes have been lacerated, but the cranial vault is intact.
3. *Penetrating:* The coverings of the brain or spinal cord have been opened.

Injuries of nervous tissue are frequently classified as follows:

1. *Concussion:* The lesions of the brain are probably variable and not readily demonstrable but always reversible. The level of consciousness varies, and even if the patient was rendered unconscious, this should clear quickly.
2. *Contusion:* There is injury to the smaller blood vessels, with minute collections of blood cells in the brain substance. The signs and symptoms will persist for a longer time than in concussion, but should clear completely.
3. *Lacerations:* The brain substance is torn either by a penetrating object including fragments of the fractured skull or shattered by the sudden motion then deceleration of the brain itself. The brain laceration may be on the side opposite to the blow (contracoup).

Diagnosis of Craniocerebral Injuries

It is extremely important to obtain the details of the accident from all eye witnesses and emergency personnel to understand the forces that may have been suffered by the patient. The level of consciousness, including the patient's awareness of time, place, and person and ability to move the extremities when he is first seen by ambulance personnel, must be carefully documented and the findings given to the personnel of the hospital where the patient is delivered.

A history of brief unconsciousness followed by lucidity and again by coma is highly suggestive of an expanding epidural or subdural blood clot that requires immediate attention. A progressive, deepening coma indicates that either a blood clot is expanding or that the traumatized brain is becoming more edematous. Unrelenting coma that was immediately present suggests severe brain damage and is an ominous sign.

The level of consciousness must be documented by recording the response of the patient to commands or painful stimuli and should be checked at regular intervals during transportation and after arrival at the emergency department. A flow sheet that includes the vital signs and the patient's responses as well as the fluids and medications administered is an important adjunct to the patient's management.

Diagnosis of Coma

The following mnemonic device, "vowel plus tips," may aid in the differential diagnosis of the cause of unconsciousness:

1. A—alcohol.
2. E—encephalopathy.
3. I—insulin.
4. O—opiates and sedatives.
5. U—uremia and metabolic.
    +
6. T—trauma,
7. I—infection (meningitis and encephalitis).
8. P—psychiatric.
9. S—syncope and seizures.

Examination

VITAL SIGNS

It must always be remembered that the brain is protected inside a bony structure. For this reason, increasing pressure from brain edema, by forcing herniation of the brainstem, can be devastating. As intracranial pressure rises, the compensatory initial response is for the pulse and respiratory rates to slow and for the blood pressure and temperature to rise. As the swelling increases, thereby reducing the blood flow and producing anoxia, compensation is lost and the pulse and respiratory rates usually become rapid and the blood pressure may fall.

	Compensated	Uncompensated
Pulse rate	↓	↑
Respiratory rate	↓	↑
Blood pressure	↑	↓
Temperature	↑	↑ ↓

EYE SIGNS

Direct damage to the eye or to the second or third cranial nerves can alter the significance of pupil changes and muscle paralysis, and the findings must be correlated with the level of consciousness.

With cortical lesions, the eyes tend to deviate to the side of the lesion. The pupils are small, but will react to light or to pain.

The normal awake person will move the eyes in the same direction as the head is turned unless the eyes have been fixed voluntarily on a point. "Doll's eyes" reflex (oculocephalic reflex), which is not normally present in conscious patients past 1 year of age, is said to be present when the eyes move in the direction opposite to which the head is turned. Doll's eyes response, when abnormally present, indicates that the frontopontine pathways are intact. The presence of the doll's eyes reflex in a comatose patient therefore indicates that the lesion is above the brainstem. In the unconscious person when the ear canal is irrigated with ice water the eyes will deviate to the same side if the brainstem pathways are intact. When the doll's eyes reflex is lost, along with loss of the response to ice water irrigation of the ear canal, the loss of brainstem function is demonstrated. Profound coma will also abolish the oculocephalic reflex as well as the caloric response.

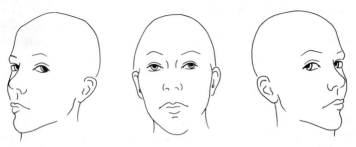

Metabolic Eye Signs
The pupils are usually small, but remain reactive to light. *Destructive lesions of the midbrain abolish this light reflex.* Acute anoxia of the brain produces pupillary constriction until the cardiac output is less than 70 percent, at which point dilation usually occurs. However, the pupils may remain small or in midposition through cardiac arrest until death.

In brainstem lesions, the eyes tend to look away from the side of the lesion. The pupils are usually fixed in midposition and are unresponsive, and there is no adjustment of the eyes to head movement. No response is obtained to ice water irrigation.

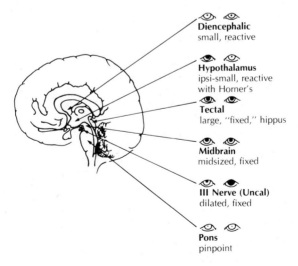

Diencephalic
small, reactive

Hypothalamus
ipsi-small, reactive
with Horner's

Tectal
large, "fixed," hippus

Midbrain
midsized, fixed

III Nerve (Uncal)
dilated, fixed

Pons
pinpoint

Central Nervous System Wounds
HEAD WOUNDS

Any indicated roentgenograms of the head or neck (or both) should be made prior to suture of scalp wounds. If the head wound is serious enough to warrant roentgenograms of the skull, the spinal column should be examined at the same time for fractures or dislocations. Cross-table views of the cervical spine must be made before moving the neck. Roentgenograms of the spine must include oblique views and especially views of C7; the latter may be better demonstrated by pulling on the arms as the film is exposed.

Minor Head Wounds

In scalp wounds, the hair should be shaved away for 2 inches around the lesion. The wound should be thoroughly irrigated with normal saline to remove any foreign material and the skin infiltrated with a local anesthetic. Then the wound is carefully explored with the gloved finger. Jagged edges and devitalized tissue are debrided and active bleeders ligated with fine silk. Further hemostasis and wound closure are achieved by closing both the galea and the skin in separate layers with interrupted sutures of fine suture material. The dressing may be held in place by sutures of 2-0 black silk that were inserted before the wound closure was started. These are tied over a bolster made by rolling up a 4 × 4 gauze sponge. The application of collodion to scalp wounds is not advised.

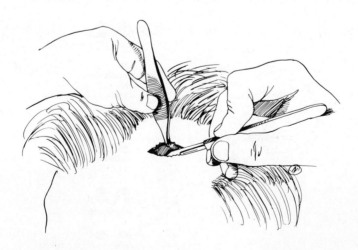

Preliminary Treatment of Major Head Wounds

Head wounds associated with signs of neurologic damage or communicating with fractures of the skull are covered with a sterile dry dressing held in place with a conforming gauze roll applied without pressure. Neurosurgical consultation should be obtained. If spinal fluid is leaking from the ear or nose, caution the patient *not* to blow his nose but to blot it with a sterile 4 × 4 gauze sponge. Cover an ear leaking spinal fluid with a sterile gauze bandage. *Do not* insert any cotton plugs.

Emergency Department Craniotomy

Most patients admitted to the emergency department in an agonal state with a history clearly compatible with an extradural hematoma may be temporarily stabilized by the intravenous administration of mannitol (1.0 to 1.5 gm per kilogram as a 20% solution in water) and transferred to the operating room. Only extremely rarely is an emergency craniotomy indicated. However, in certain circumstances it may be necessary to immediately relieve the pressure in order to keep the patient alive so that he can be transferred.

The temporal area is shaved and prepared, although this may be omitted if time is lacking. The skin incision is made 2 cm anterior to the ear and extending upward from the zygomatic arch for 5 cm. The skin and muscles may be held apart with a small self-retaining retractor such as a mastoid retractor.

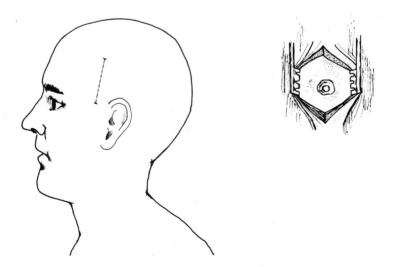

A small drill is used to make a hole in the thin temporal bone to allow the blood to escape. A dressing of dry gauze is applied with a conforming bandage, and the patient is transferred to the operating room of the receiving hospital.

Management of Suspected Vertebral Column Injury

Patients who arrive at the hospital with possible injuries of the vertebral column that are not splinted should be strapped to a backboard or have a head halter applied, or both, before any manipulations or examinations are carried out.

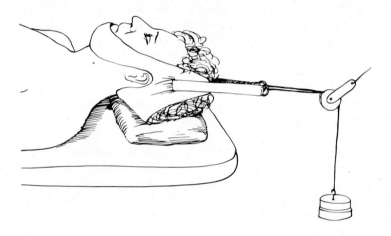

INSERTION OF CRUTCHFIELD TONGS

Tongs are inserted in any case of a fracture of the cervical verte-brae with or without any evidence of neurologic damage. The skin is shaved and prepared over the indicated skin sites in line with the mastoid processes. The tongs are centered over the skull, and the points are used to indent and mark the skin. The skin is incised with a stab-bladed knife, and a drill with a guarded tip is used to make the hole only in the outer table of the skull.

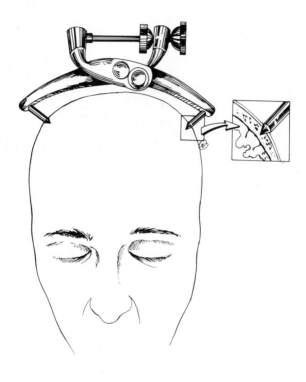

A rope connects the tongs over a pulley at the head of the bed and is connected to weights. Weights of 5 to 15 pounds are used for children and weights of 10 to 50 pounds for adults. The weight will depend on the size and response of the fracture or dislocation (or both). The head end of the bed should be elevated approximately 10° to allow the patient's body weight to act as countertraction. The tongs and traction system must be inspected and adjusted daily to ensure against slippage.

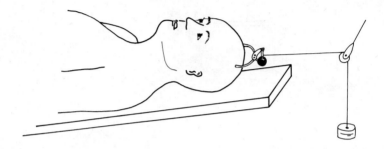

Tongs designed by Dr. James Gardner and called Gardner-Wells tongs are also available. They may be inserted without shaving any hair. The pins are sharp and approach the skull at an upward angle when inserted through the temporal muscle several centimeters above the ear. The main disadvantage of these tongs for long-term use is limitation of head rotation, since the pins on the metal arc protrude far to the sides. However, they are ideal for immediate use and, when properly applied, have less tendency to slip out than do Crutchfield tongs, which approach the top of the skull at an oblique, downward angle.

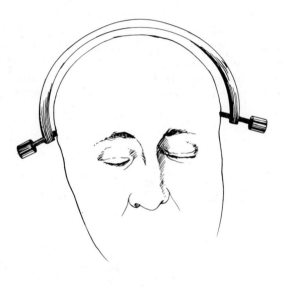

Peripheral Nerve Repair

Suturing of peripheral nerves should be done only under optimal conditions by physicians experienced in the technique. If the wound is more than 6 hours old or is dirty, or other untoward conditions exist, it is cleaned by thorough saline irrigation and removal of any devitalized or foreign material. The skin edges are then debrided and closed, anticipating later repair of the nerve or nerves.

Approximate the nerve ends without tension. Align nerve ends, identifying the proximal and distal ends of surface blood vessels. Place a marking suture in the sheath only. Using a razor blade, recut the damaged ends. Reapproximate the ends by interrupted sutures of 7-0 atraumatic material that catch only the nerve sheath. The suture is usually lubricated by running the needle and suture through fat. The skin is closed in the usual fashion, and the extremity is splinted so as to avoid tension on the anastomosis.

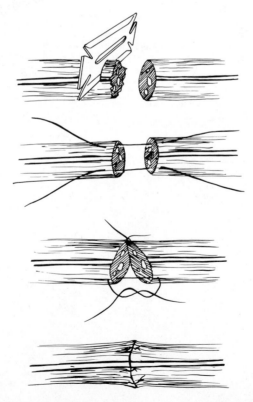

Lumbar Puncture

A lumbar puncture set includes the following:

1. Manometer.
2. Needles, 22- and 25-gauge, 1½ inches in length.
3. Spinal needles, 20- and 22-gauge.
4. Three-way stopcock.
5. Culture and collecting tubes.
6. Ampules of anesthetic.
7. "Prep" set.
8. Gloves.

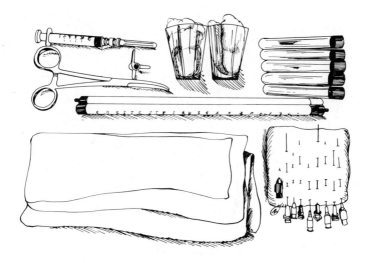

A lumbar puncture must not be done in any patient with suspected increased intracranial pressure.

The patient is held firmly on his side by an assistant with the spinal column flexed. The back is prepared and a wheal of local anesthetic is raised in the skin. The anesthetic is then infiltrated between the third and fourth lumbar interspaces including the spinous interspace (level of posterior superior spine of the iliac crests).

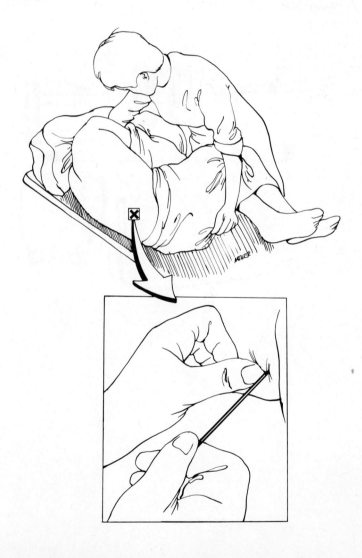

The spinal needle is inserted, perpendicular to the sagittal plane and inclined 30° cephalad. When the ligamentum flavum is passed, a "give" will be felt, and the stylette is removed. If no spinal fluid is obtained, the needle is rotated and may be advanced carefully without the stylette. If bone is encountered in the subcutaneous area, the needle is probably striking the spinous process and should be angled more cephalad. If bone is encountered at a greater depth, the needle may be striking a facet and should be redirected more caudad.

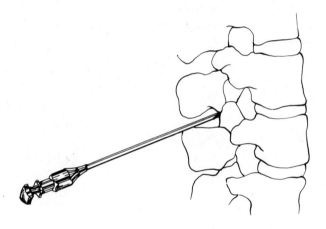

Cisternal Tap (Infants)

Cisternal tap may be performed on an infant or child to relieve increased intracranial pressure or for diagnostic purposes if fluid cannot be obtained by lumbar puncture. The back of the neck is shaved and prepared. The child is held rigidly with the head acutely flexed on the chest.

The needle is introduced at the base of the skull at a point on a line through the auditory meatus and the glabella of the nose. The insertion point may be infiltrated with a local anesthetic. The needle should penetrate no more than 1.5 to 2 cm. As the needle is passed, the stylette should be removed frequently until spinal fluid is obtained.

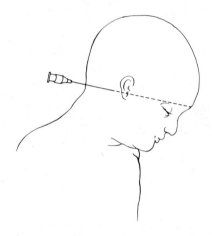

An alternative approach is lateral cervical canal puncture between the laminae of C1 and C2. This should only be done with fluoroscopic or x-ray control to guide the needle precisely and avoid entry into neural tissue.

Subdural Tap

A subdural tap can be easily performed in an infant for diagnosis or to remove a collection of blood. The infant must be completely restrained on a board or by a sheet, and the head is fixed by a nurse with a hand on each side. The scalp and the fontanelles are carefully palpated to find the coronal suture. This area of the scalp is shaved, prepared, and anesthetized.

The operator's nondominant hand rests on the child's head and braces the needle, which is introduced by the dominant hand. The needle is inserted into the coronal suture just lateral to the anterior fontanelle at least 3 cm from the midline. As the dura is passed, there will be a sudden lessening of resistance to passage of the needle. If blood is found, the tap should be repeated on the opposite side of the skull. Repeated daily taps may be performed to relieve excessive pressure on the brain.

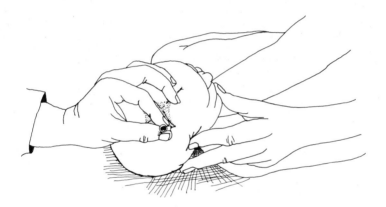

8

Management of Outpatient Problems of the Head and Neck

Donald G. Sessions

Examination
Examination of the face and neck is primarily performed by observation, palpation, and auscultation.

OBSERVATION
The most important point in examination of the face and neck is the presence or absence of symmetry of the two sides. The ears, eyes, nostrils, lips, and both sides of the neck are normally symmetrical. The pupils are ordinarily at the same planar level. Indentations or protrusions, lumps and masses, decreased movement, or paralysis are all abnormalities. The motion of the mandible in opening and closing is normally symmetrical and midline.

PALPATION
Palpation of the face and neck is bimanual. The skull, cricoid area, supraorbital and infraorbital rims, nose, mandible, and neck are all felt with gentle thoroughness. Bimanual palpation of the floor of the mouth (A) and the base of the tongue (B) is shown. The areas of frequent injury include the malar eminence, infraorbital rim, nasal bones, and mandible. The larynx is palpated in its relationship to the hyoid bone and the cricoid cartilage. Special attention is paid to determining the presence or absence of crepitance as a sign of air in the soft tissues. This gives a standard "Rice Krispy" feeling.

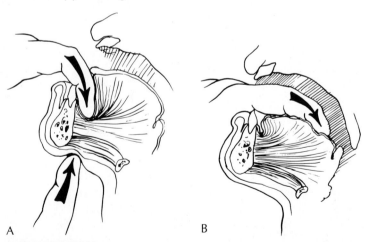

A   B

AUSCULTATION
Auscultation of the face and neck is used to determine whether or not vascular lesions, particularly traumatic arteriovenous fistulas, are present.

Local Anesthesia

Local anesthesia of the face and neck includes local and topical blocks of the ear, nose, mandible, maxilla, and neck. Most traumatic lesions of the face and neck lend themselves to successful repair under local anesthesia.

TECHNIQUE

Ear

PINNA. Several injections of 1% local anesthetic into the soft tissue in the sulcus behind the ear will satisfactorily anesthetize the entire pinna.

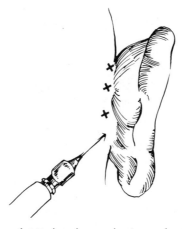

CANAL. Injection of 1% local anesthetic at the junction of the bony and cartilaginous ear canal in four quadrants will adequately anesthetize the ear canal and tympanic membrane for such procedures as foreign body removal or myringotomy.

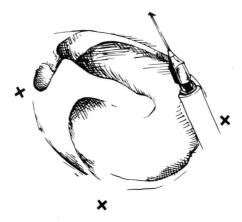

Nose

In patients over the age of 15 years, local anesthetic can be used successfully for almost any nasal procedure. After satisfactory skin preparation, cocaine flakes are topically applied to two main areas of the nasal mucous membrane with cotton-tipped metal application sticks: (1) high in the superior meatus to block the branches of the nasociliary nerve; (2) posteriorly in the middle meatus to block the branches of the sphenopalatine ganglion.

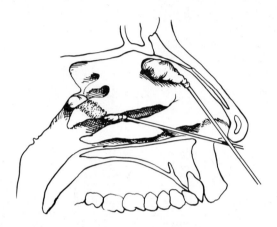

While the topical anesthetic is working, 1% lidocaine (Xylocaine) with 1:200,000 epinephrine is injected bilaterally in the following areas:

1. From a point just lateral to the ala:
   a. The infraorbital nerve is blocked where it comes out of the infraorbital foramen with a long needle.
   b. The infratrochlear nerves are blocked using a long needle just lateral to the nasion.
   c. The anterior alveolar nerves are blocked near the anterior nasal spine.

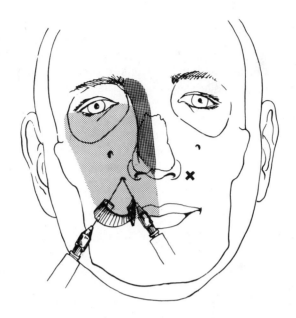

2. Through the nostril:
   a. The needle enters just above the rim of the upper lateral cartilage and continues upward over the lateral portion of the nasal bone. Anesthetic is deposited as the needle is withdrawn.
   b. More anesthetic is then injected into the membranous nasal septum itself and again into the area of the nasal spine.

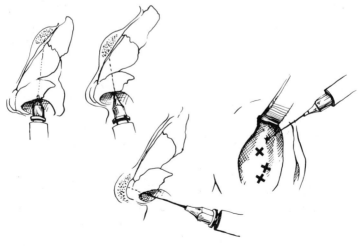

Mandible

A complete block of mandibular sensation may be produced by injection into the mandibular sulcus on the inner surface of the ramus. This blocks the inferior alveolar, lingual, and long buccal nerves. The retromolar trigone is palpated with the mouth partially open (A). The needle is inserted at the apex of the pterygo-mandibular raphe and advanced between the ramus and the ligaments and muscles covering the internal surface until the point is felt against the posterior wall (B). About 2 ml of anesthetic is deposited here and another milliliter is injected while withdrawing the needle along the point of insertion.

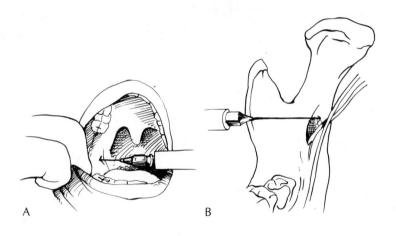

A   B

Maxilla

The posterior superior alveolar nerve is blocked by injecting anesthetic above the third molar on the zygomatic aspect of the maxilla. The infraorbital nerve is blocked as previously described. The nasopalatine nerve is blocked by injecting anesthetic in the region of the midline anterior palatine canal. This provides anesthesia to the anterior third of the palate. The greater palatine nerve is blocked by injecting the greater palatine foramen, which is palpable just medial to the third molar. This provides anesthesia to the posterior two-thirds of the palate.

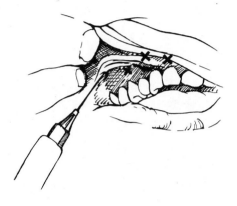

Neck

LOCAL AREAS. Local infiltration of the neck is satisfactory for minor excisional work as well as for functional procedures such as tracheostomy.

CERVICAL BLOCK. Cervical block is used for procedures on deeper structures of the neck. This should not be done on an outpatient basis.

Traumatic Lesions of the Face
SOFT TISSUE WOUNDS

Soft tissue wounds constitute a large proportion of facial injuries and vary from simple, clean lacerations to ragged, crushed wounds grossly contaminated with dirt and foreign bodies with extensive loss of tissue.

Examination

Observation for the extent of injury includes:

1. Neural injuries.
2. Muscular weakness.
3. Salivary duct function.
4. Presence or absence of a foreign body.
5. Possible underlying fractures.

Palpation for masses, fracture, crepitance, and foreign bodies is carried out, and roentgenograms are taken.

Treatment

Pretreatment photographs of the injury may be taken. In treatment, the basic principle to be followed is strict conservation of all wounded tissue, including mucous membranes, bone, muscle, subcutaneous tissue, and skin. No tissue that is viable should be sacrificed. Mechanical cleansing takes the place of debridement. The wound is thoroughly explored and irrigated with saline, and hemostasis is attained.

Primary closure is desirable. Any wound with areas of deep involvement below the skin and subcutaneous tissue or with nerve or salivary duct involvement should be closed in an operating room.

Laceration of the Lips

TREATMENT: GENERAL. The position and movement of the lips are important factors in facial expression. Surgeons should make every effort to obtain a satisfactory cosmetic result in treating injuries to this area. The lips have a rich vascular supply from the superior and inferior labial arteries of the external carotid system. Ischemia or necrosis is seldom a surgical complication in this site.

In repair of wounds of the lips the single most important problem is the accurate approximation of the vermilion border. Breaks or notches in the usual smooth sharp line of the vermilion border are noticeable and call attention to other scars in the region.

Simple uncomplicated through-and-through lacerations of the lip can be closed on an outpatient basis. Patients with jagged, dirty, or otherwise complicated lacerations of the lip should be admitted to the hospital, as should patients with tissue loss requiring flap rotation.

TECHNIQUE OF CLOSURE. Following gentle but thorough mechanical cleansing of the wound (A) with white soap (B) and irrigation with normal saline (C), the lip is anesthetized by local infiltration anesthesia with 1% lidocaine. Marks are then made along the vermilion-skin junction with methylene blue dye on a pointed applicator. Layered closure of the muscle, subcutaneous tissue, and skin is then accomplished (D, E). The muscle layer is approximated with 3-0 chromic catgut and the skin and mucosa with 5-0 nylon interrupted sutures. Special attention is made to evert the closure at the vermilion border slightly to prevent future notching.

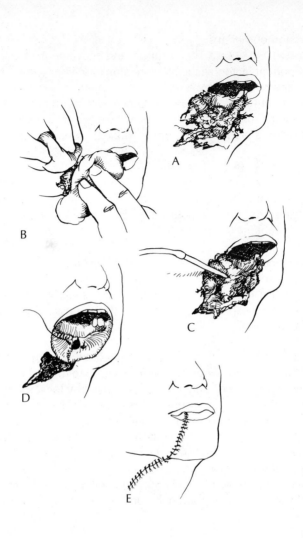

A

B

C

D

E

Lacerations of the Mouth

Simple lacerations of the soft palate, buccal mucosa, floor of the mouth, and tongue are readily treated on an outpatient basis. Patients with complicated oral and orapharyngeal injuries should be admitted to the hospital. Through-and-through lacerations of the soft palate should be treated in an operating room. The blood supply of these areas is excellent, and outpatient suture of these lacerations is predominantly for hemostasis rather than for functional benefit. After the injection of 1% lidocaine, lacerations of the tongue or buccal mucosa are sutured into previous anatomic balance with 3-0 chromic catgut. Because of continued mobility the tongue sutures can be expected to slough by day 2 or 3, but hemostasis is usually satisfactory by that time.

BONY INJURIES

Almost any severe trauma to the face results in a fracture because of the exposed position of the facial bones and minimal soft tissue protection. Single bone fracture is rare, and a combination of fractures of facial bones is common.

Nasal Fracture

Trauma to the nose is the most common facial injury. It may involve the skin, soft tissue over the nose, nasal bones, frontal process of the maxilla, the cartilages, and the nasal septum. The nasal bones may be displaced in an antero-posterior direction or laterally.

EXAMINATION. Fracture of the nasal bones is diagnosed by observation and palpation, when swelling and asymmetry are noted. Intranasal examination is mandatory to diagnose mucosal lacerations or septal deformities.

TREATMENT: GENERAL. Simple nasal fractures of recent origin can be readily treated on an outpatient basis. Patients with more complicated nasal fractures, including those combined with soft tissue injury or other facial bone injuries, should be admitted to the hospital. Lacerations about the nose should receive initial attention. Following wound cleansing the wound is sutured so that all anatomic relationships are maintained; 5-0 nylon suture is employed.

TECHNIQUE FOR REDUCTION OF NASAL FRACTURE. Following skin cleansing, a topical and local anesthetic is applied as previously described. Simple fractures (A) are realigned with a blunt, wide scalpel handle inserted underneath the depressed nasal bones intranasally (B). Outward pressure against the bone moves it into position. A finger on the outer surface of the nose directs and controls the position of the fragment (C). The displaced nasal walls are thus elevated and molded into position bimanually. Attention must always be directed to the correction of obstructing bony or cartilaginous nasal septum, which can be straightened into the midline with an Ash or Walsham forceps (D). Intranasal packing will hold the bony fragments in proper position. An external tape and metal splint is then applied.

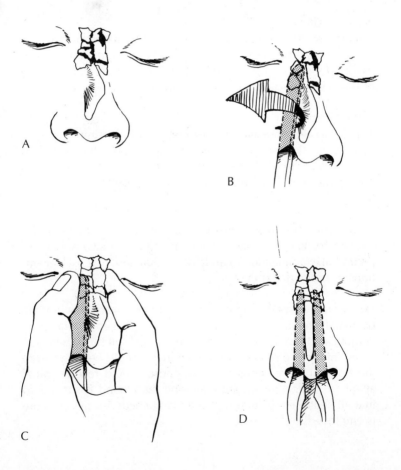

Fracture of the Mandible

Second to the nose, the mandible is the most commonly fractured bone of the face. The most common area of fracture is the mandibular body in the region of the molar teeth or near the mental foramen. A fracture of the body is often associated with a fracture of the contralateral condyle. Bilateral condyle fractures are common.

EXAMINATION. A diagnosis of mandibular fracture is made by observing areas of abnormal mobility, hemorrhage, and tenderness. There is loss of normal dental occlusion, and an open bite deformity is common.

ROENTGENOGRAMS. Standard films of the mandible should include views of the body, symphysis, and condyle on each side. Panorex view of the mandible is especially valuable.

TREATMENT: GENERAL. Provide an adequate airway by traction of the mandible forward and upward. Dentitious mandible fractures are "open" fractures and patients with such fractures are placed on antibiotics. Reduction and immobilization of simple fractures of the mandible in dentulous patients can be readily performed on an outpatient basis. The standard treatment for this type of injury is the application of arch bars and interdental wiring under local anesthesia.

TECHNIQUE OF APPLICATION OF ARCH BARS. Local anesthesia to the mandible and maxilla is given as previously described. A pre-formed arch bar is wired to the teeth of the mandible and maxilla with No. 24 stainless steel wires. Wire is placed around each tooth except the central incisors. Reduction is accomplished by rubber bands placed between the two arch bars, which pull the bones into position. The rubber bands may be replaced by wire after the fracture is reduced.

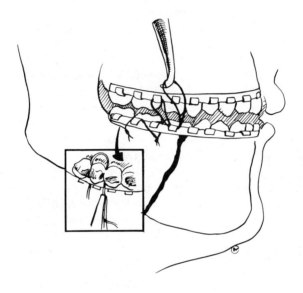

Postreduction x-ray films are taken to assure reduction. Dental care during immobilization is necessary and is aided by the use of a Water-Pik. The diet is liquid and should be supplemental. The wires and arch bars are left on for between 4 and 6 weeks.

Patients with complicated fractures and edentulous patients with fractures should be admitted to the hospital for definitive care.

Fracture of the Zygoma

Fractures of the zygoma are sometimes overlooked because of overlying swelling, which may hide the cosmetic deformity. Although these fractures may be simple, most fractures of the zygoma involve the neighboring maxilla, temporal, and frontal bones.

EXAMINATION. Observation reveals ecchymosis, subconjunctival hemorrhage, depression of the malar eminence, and downward displacement of the eye. Palpation reveals fractures, especially of the orbital rim. Diplopia may mean significant entrapment of eye muscles. Complete ophthalmologic evaluation is mandatory. Numbness of the face may indicate fracture through the infraorbital foramen.

TREATMENT. Definitive treatment of these fractures should be carried out in the hospital.

Midface Fractures

Midface fractures are complicated injuries that usually involve both sides of the face. Hemorrhage from the nose and pharynx may occur. Early respiratory obstruction is often present, and cerebral injury is frequently associated. Severe facial deformities are the most common presenting symptoms.

EXAMINATION. Examination of a patient with a midface fracture is made by observation of the face. Severe swelling is present. The entire middle portion of the face may be pushed inward, giving a severely flattened appearance. There is often loss of normal occlusion.

On palpation, abnormal mobility is found when impaction has not occurred, and the maxillary alveolus or the entire face can often be moved forward and backward as well as up and down. Palpation of the orbital rims may reveal palpable fractures. Nasal bone fractures may be palpated. Numbness of the upper face usually suggests fracture through the infraorbital foramina.

ROENTGENOGRAMS. Standard facial films are taken to include the stereo-Waters view, the lateral view, the Caldwell view, and the submental vertical view. Skull films should be included because of the high incidence of associated cranial injury.

TREATMENT. Emergency treatment is usually aimed at stopping acute hemorrhage and obtaining a satisfactory airway. After the patient's condition is stabilized, photographs are taken, and the patient is admitted to the hospital for definitive treatment.

Dislocations of the Mandible

Dislocation of the condyle of the mandible from the glenoid fossa may occur either unilaterally or bilaterally when the mouth is opened wide or when the joint is subjected to sudden trauma. The condyle is pushed over the articular tubercle into the zygomatic fossa. The mandible then becomes fixed in this position as a result of the contracture of the elevator muscles of the jaws.

EXAMINATION. The mandible is fixed in abnormal position downward and locked open. The patient cannot close the mouth. Roentgenograms reveal the condyle of the mandible dislocated anterior to the articular eminence of the glenoid fossa.

TREATMENT. To reduce the dislocation, the fingers of both hands are placed beneath the jaw, and the thumbs are placed in the mouth on the occlusal surfaces of the mandibular molars. It is wise to protect the thumbs with gauze pads wrapped around them. Pressure is exerted in a downward and posterior direction, and the dislocated condyle usually slides into the glenoid fossa. Sedatives and analgesics are sometimes required. When severe trismus resists mandibular motion, the dislocation sometimes requires injection of local anesthetic into the joint and sometimes even general anesthesia.

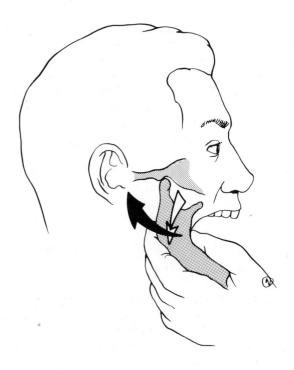

Infections of the Head
SINUS
Acute Maxillary Sinusitis
Symptoms of sinus infection include pain over the sinus, headaches, tenderness on pressure, and olfactory disturbances.

EXAMINATION. Objective signs of acute maxillary sinusitis include swelling and edema, nasal discharge, and pus in the nasopharynx.

ROENTGENOGRAMS. Standard sinus films include stereo-Waters, lateral, Caldwell, and submental vertical views. Acute sinusitis presents either as membrane thickening, air-fluid level, or partial or complete opacification.

TREATMENT. After appropriate cultures of the nose, treatment of acute sinusitis requires antibiotics, decongestants, humidification of the air, and analgesics to alleviate the pain. Local measures to decrease edema and inflammation in the nose are often useful. These include Neo-Synephrine nasal spray and liquid ephedrine or cocaine-soaked cotton pledgets placed in each nasal meatus on applicator sticks. Irrigation of the maxillary sinuses is not ordinarily done when the patient has an acute infection.

Frontal Sinusitis

EXAMINATION. Most patients with acute frontal sinusitis appear ill. They have a severe headache and are toxic. Tenderness to palpation of the floor of the frontal sinus on the affected side is present.

ROENTGENOGRAMS. X-ray films reveal opacification or air-fluid level in the frontal sinus and sometimes in associated sinuses.

TREATMENT. Frontal sinusitis is treated as a severe life-threatening illness. Following culture of the nose and standard blood cultures, the patient is placed on high doses of antibiotics and decongestants. Local measures are applied. The patient is usually admitted to the hospital. Absolute indications for hospital admission of patients with acute frontal sinusitis include the following: (1) signs of intracranial extension of infection, such as meningitis, subdural abscess, or brain abscess; (2) persistent pain that has not responded to adequate conservative therapy; (3) necrosis of the sinus wall; (4) mucocele on sinus x-ray examination; (5) orbital cellulitis with abscess formation or retrobulbar neuritis.

Irrigation of the frontal sinus for acute infection is not technically feasible and is contraindicated. Drainage of a frontal sinus through a trephine operation is an inpatient procedure.

FACE

Infections of the face, particularly around the nose, are treated with great vigor because of the danger of extension of the infection into deeper areas. The veins of the face do not have valves, and retrograde extension of infection from the angular vein lateral to the nose can result in meningitis or cavernous sinus thrombosis.

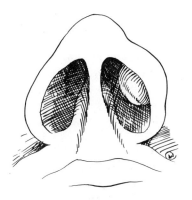

Examination

Observations of the area of involvement should be supplemented by examination of the nose and nasopharynx with a nasal speculum after shrinking the nasal mucous membranes with Neo-Synephrine spray. The nasopharynx must be examined with a mirror. Ophthalmologic evaluation is mandatory.

Associated signs, including orbital cellulitis, edema of the optic disc, ophthalmoplegia, or meningeal signs may indicate cavernous sinus thrombosis. Roentgenograms of the sinuses may reveal underlying sinus infection.

Treatment

The patient should be admitted to the hospital if any signs of toxicity are present. Appropriate cultures are taken, and high-dose antibiotics against gram-positive organisms are begun intravenously. Associated signs, including orbital cellulitis, edema of the optic disc, or meningeal signs, may indicate cavernous sinus thrombosis, and the patient should be hospitalized.

ACUTE TONSILLITIS
Patients with acute tonsillitis are usually toxic, with high fever, severe sore throat, and difficulty in swallowing.

Examination
Tonsils are red, swollen, and covered with yellow spots of exudate. Acute tonsillitis should be differentiated from nonbacterial pharyngitis, infectious mononucleosis, and occasionally diphtheria.

Treatment
The pharynx is cultured. Antibiotic treatment is given predominantly for gram-positive organisms, usually group A beta-hemolytic streptococci. Penicillin or erythromycin are commonly given. Warm saline mouth washes bring symptomatic relief. Bed rest and forcing fluids are employed when patients are toxic.

PERITONSILLAR ABSCESS
In most cases of peritonsillar abscess the pus has broken through into the supratonsillar fossa. There is marked swelling and edema of the soft palate to the extent that the tonsil is pushed downward and medially. Penetration deep to the superior constrictor muscle allows pus into the parapharyngeal space. Pus in this space may descend into the neck or mediastinum. Symptoms include fever, toxicity, sore throat, and difficulty in swallowing.

Examination
Trismus on examination is an indication of encroachment of the muscles of mastication by the abscess. Torticollis is an indication of infiltration of tissue of the neck. There is usually marked asymmetrical swelling of the tonsil and soft palate on the involved side. Digital examination of the tonsillar region may reveal fluctuation. Roentgenograms may show pus in the parapharyngeal space.

Treatment: General

Antipyretics, analgesics, and antibiotics should be given, and warm saline gargles are begun. If fluctuation is present or pus in the deeper tissues is indicated, incision and drainage of the abscess is considered. A small accumulation of palpable pus in the supratonsillar fossa can be incised and drained on an outpatient basis. However, most children, as well as patients with indications of deep extension of pus, including trismus or torticollis, should be admitted to the hospital for the procedure.

Technique of Incision and Drainage

Injection of 1% lidocaine into the region of the incision results in local anesthesia. The point of incision is important. An imaginary horizontal line is made from the point on the contralateral or normal side where the anterior-posterior pillars meet the beginning of the uvula. A vertical line is drawn just in front of the anterior pillar on the side of involvement. The incision is made where these two lines bisect and is carried beyond the outer border of the tonsil and deep. At least two suction apparatuses should be available so that the pus will not cause aspiration or other complications.

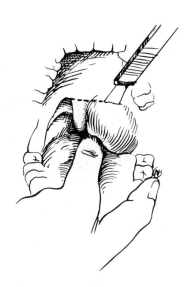

Close follow-up is important, and the tonsils should usually be removed electively following an abscess.

RETROPHARYNGEAL ABSCESS

Retropharyngeal abscesses are due to suppuration from (1) retro-pharyngeal nodes, (2) posterior pharyngeal wall infection, (3) foreign body, (4) extension of infection from the ear, and (5) extension of infection from the parotid gland.

Examination

The patient has a sore throat, pain on swallowing, and signs of respiratory obstruction. There is fluctuant swelling of the retro-pharyngeal area (usually unilateral). Palpation of the mass shows no pulsation and differentiates the mass from an aneurysm of the internal carotid artery. Roentgenograms of the neck reveal the mass in the retropharynx.

Treatment: General

The airway is secured, and antibiotics and warm saline gargles are begun. The abscess should be incised and drained.

Technique for Incision and Drainage

Small, high abscesses can be drained transorally under local anesthesia on an outpatient basis.

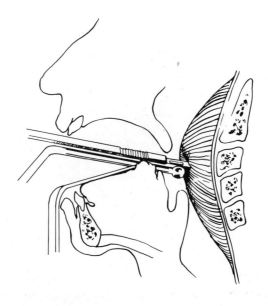

Deeper retropharyngeal abscesses with inferior extension require admission to the hospital for open neck exploration under general anesthesia. The incision is made anterior to the carotid sheath and carried deep to the retropharyngeal area for dependent drainage.

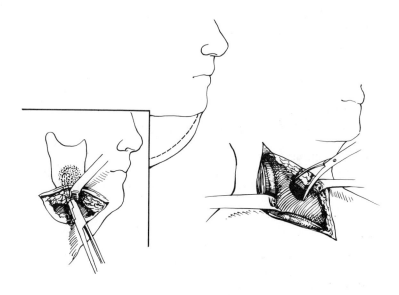

INFECTIONS OF THE FLOOR OF THE MOUTH
Infections of the floor of the mouth, or Ludwig's angina, may become a serious problem. Any infection of the floor of the mouth is liable by edema to encroach seriously on the pharynx and supraglottis and thus on the airway.

Examination
A firm swelling of the submandibular and submental areas with induration of the floor of the mouth, gums, and tongue is seen on examination. The tongue is pushed upward and backward. Trismus may be present.

Treatment
Antibiotics and warm saline soaks are started. Tracheostomy must be considered in the presence of any degree of respiratory obstruction. Patients with fluctuance or signs of extension of pus such as trismus should be admitted for definitive therapy, including incision and drainage.

Foreign Bodies in the Nose

EXAMINATION

Symptoms of nasal foreign body include signs of acute sinusitis, profuse unilateral mucopurulent discharge of long duration, pain, and headache. Most of the patients will either be young children or patients with psychiatric problems.

TECHNIQUE OF REMOVAL OF NASAL FOREIGN BODY

No Anesthesia

Young children may be gently secured by wrapping them in sheets in the standard fashion. The nose is then sprayed with Neo-Synephrine. A standard foreign body forceps must be used to remove foreign bodies. A curved probe should be used to get behind round foreign objects such as beads or marbles.

Local Anesthesia

In older children and adults, a local or a general anesthetic may be needed. This may require admission to the hospital.

Epistaxis

Epistaxis, or bleeding from the interior of the nose, may be spontaneous or induced. Hemorrhage may come from the anterior part of the nasal septum (Kiesselbach's, or Little's, area) or from more posterior areas of the nose.

CAUSES

It is important to take a brief history to determine the cause of the nosebleed. Common causes of nosebleed that may require more than local treatment include trauma, a recent surgical procedure, high blood pressure, blood dyscrasia or coagulation defects, and medications or drugs, especially anticoagulants.

EXAMINATION

Accurate localization of the site of the bleeding is important because posterior superior bleeders are supplied by the ethmoid arteries of the internal carotid system, and the remainder of the nose is supplied by the branches of the sphenopalatine artery of the external carotid system.

TREATMENT

Obtaining vital signs and the determination of the hematocrit will help gauge the amount of blood loss secondary to hemorrhage. Blood for replacement is typed and crossed-matched immediately.

Attention is directed to stopping the bleeding. Use of the headlight or head mirror with suction apparatus allows the physician to clean the nose and attempt to find the exact site of bleeding. A metal nasal suction tube (No. 10 Frazier) is used.

ANTERIOR EPISTAXIS

A small bleeder on the membranous nasal septum can be cauterized with a silver nitrate stick. A vigorous bleeder on the membranous septum sometimes requires cotton packs impregnated with Borofax ointment. Bleeding from a more posterior point will require widespread anterior packing of the nose. This is performed by inserting ½-inch Vaseline gauze in the middle meatus and working forward and downward until the entire inferior meatus is filled. Gauze is then worked superiorly, and finally the middle meatus is filled with the gauze. The posterior end of the pack must extend to the posterior choana. Anterior nasal packing should be left in place for at least 48 hours. Occasionally, patients with anterior packing must be admitted for observation, but most may be discharged home to bed rest.

POSTERIOR EPISTAXIS

When standard anterior nasal packing does not control the bleeding, posterior packing is used. This can be done readily in the outpatient area.

Using headlight illumination, metal suction tubing, and a nasal speculum and with the patient in a sitting position, the nose and nasopharynx are shrunk down as much as possible with 0.25% Neo-Synephrine; this may be contraindicated in patients with high blood pressure. A No. 14 Foley catheter with a 30-cc balloon is inserted on the side of the most active bleeding (A). This is inserted through the nose into the oropharynx, and about 15 cc of air is inserted into the balloon. The catheter is then retracted back into the posterior choana. If this does not stop the posterior hemorrhage, the procedure is repeated on the contralateral side. While anterior pressure is maintained on the catheter, an anterior pack is then inserted intranasally around the catheter (B). Anterior traction is maintained by the use of a screw clamp placed on the catheter over soft sponge rubber. The patient is then admitted to the hospital. The packs stay in place a minimum of 3 to 5 days.

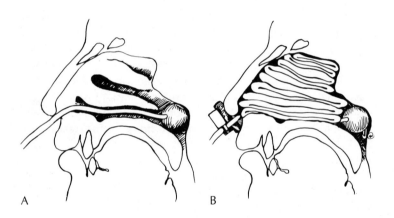

A   B

Neoplasms of the Oral Cavity

Patients with any lesion suggestive of possible malignancy should be referred to the physician who will be taking definitive care of the problem.

Cystic lesions of the floor of the mouth (ranulas), although benign, are difficult to manage and should not be incised and drained unless there are signs of infection and abscess formation. These lesions should be treated on an inpatient basis by elective marsupialization or excision.

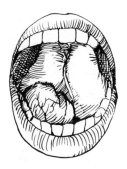

Obviously benign lesions of the tongue (A) or buccal surface (B), including epulis or papilloma, may be excised on an outpatient basis under local infiltration with 1% lidocaine anesthesia. The resultant minimal defect may be closed with 3-0 chromic catgut sutures. All tissue that is removed is sent for pathologic examination.

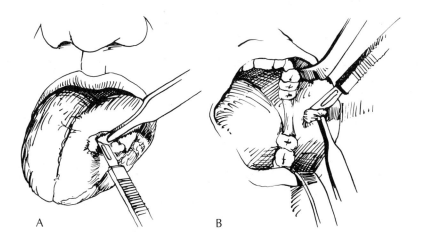

A   B

Dental Emergencies

Most patients who are seen in an emergency room setting for a dental emergency have either inflammation, hemorrhage, or trauma.

INFLAMMATION

Inflammation and infection may involve either the pulp of the tooth, the periapical area, or the periodontal structures.

Examination

The area around the tooth or teeth is red, swollen, and tender. The pus may have broken into the soft tissues of the neck, resulting in large amounts of swelling. Dental and mandibular films, including Panorex, help with the diagnosis.

Treatment

Treatment for uncomplicated infections of specific teeth includes (1) analgesics, (2) warm saline soaks, (3) antibiotics, and (4) referral to a dentist for drainage.

Patients with dental abscesses with extension of the infection beyond the teeth including cervical abscesses should be admitted to the hospital for definitive treatment.

HEMORRHAGE

Examination

Patients with recent extractions may arrive in the emergency room with acute hemorrhage from the area. Localization of the bleeding point is usually no problem.

Treatment

Pressure on the bleeding area with gauze will usually stop the hemorrhage. Injection of local anesthetic with epinephrine may be of value. Suture of elevated gingivae over the bleeding alveolus is rarely necessary.

TRAUMA

Patients with uncomplicated trauma to the teeth, not including the mandible, should be given analgesics and referred to their dentist for definitive treatment. Those with dental trauma associated with facial fractures should be admitted to the hospital for definitive care.

Ear

EXAMINATION

The external ear is examined by meticulous observation and gentle palpation. Examination of the ear canal requires the use of an ear speculum. An electric otoscope is suitable, but a head mirror is preferable because it leaves both hands free for instrumentation. The largest speculum that can be introduced without pain should be used. Time should be taken to remove cerumen or epidermal debris gently using special ear instruments. No ear examination is complete until a magnifying pneumatic otoscope is used to delineate the status of the tympanic membrane, including mobility, and the presence of fluid in the tympanic cavity. An operating microscope will allow inspection of the ear under satisfactory high power with maximal safety.

EXTERNAL EAR

Trauma: Aural Hematoma

Trauma to the external ear may result in contusion, laceration, or hematoma. Following severe injury, blood collects rapidly, dissecting the perichondrium and the cartilage and resulting in an aural hematoma.

EXAMINATION. Examination reveals a bluish swelling, usually involving the entire auricle. The swelling is usually fluctuant and may be tender.

TREATMENT. Early evacuation of the collected blood is essential to prevent the formation of a scarred or cauliflower ear. Aseptic surgical technique is required because of the possibility of perichondritis. Antibiotics are given. The incision should be placed in the skin parallel to the helix. Sufficient exposure should be attained to aspirate the entire hematoma. Rubber-band drains may be used to prevent the reaccumulation of blood or serum. A tight pressure dressing is placed, and the patient is seen daily for at least 5 days.

Frostbite
Frostbite of the ear indicates cold injury in which actual freezing of tissue with ice-crystal formation has occurred.

EXAMINATION. The ear may be hard and white. There may be a hyperemic line of demarcation between frozen and unfrozen tissue.

TREATMENT. The following method of treatment is proposed for treating the frozen ear:

1. Rapid rewarming with warm, wet sterile cotton pledgets at 100 to 108° F.
2. Sedatives and analgesics.
3. Sterile precautions—no dressings.
4. Antibiotics are used for deep infections only.
5. Superficial infections are treated with 0.5% silver nitrate soaks or Betadine solution.
6. No surgical debridement should be done initially.
7. No smoking.

Perichondritis
Perichondritis of the external ear is seen after trauma with infected hematoma or after ear surgery.

EXAMINATION. On examination, painful diffuse red swelling of the external ear is seen. Edema may have spread to the postauricular region, causing the auricle to protrude.

TREATMENT. Treatment of perichondritis is difficult because the usual infecting organism is often resistant. Antibiotics are given after cultures and sensitivity testing. Warm saline soaks are prescribed. Admission to the hospital for incision and drainage is often necessary.

EXTERNAL AUDITORY CANAL
Cerumen Impaction

TECHNIQUE OF CERUMEN REMOVAL. Impacted cerumen may be softened before removal with the use of half-strength hydrogen peroxide or Cerumenex. Impacted cerumen may be removed by irrigation, instrumentation, or both.

Irrigation (A) is the most gentle way of cleaning the external ear canal. A syringe or pressure-driven irrigating bottle is used to irrigate the external ear canal gently. Under direct visualization the water stream is directed along the superior canal wall so that the returning stream may push the cerumen from behind. The outflow is caught in a basin held tightly below the ear.

A cerumen curette will sometimes allow removal of firm wax. A middle ear forceps is used to remove firm wax gently (B). A cotton-tipped metal applicator may be used to remove softer wax gently. Suction is used to remove moist cerumen and to dry the canal (C).

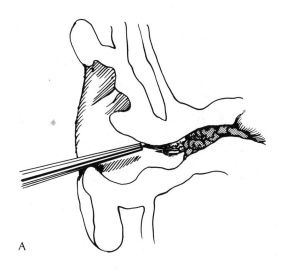

A

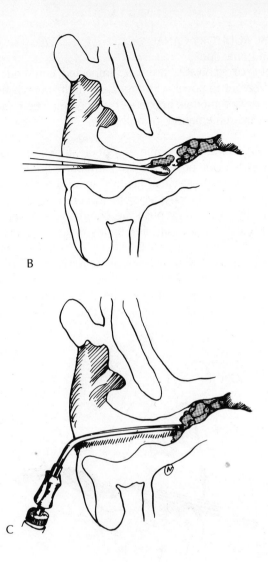

B

C

Foreign Bodies

TECHNIQUE OF FOREIGN BODY REMOVAL. Removing a foreign body from the external ear canal requires delicate technique and gentleness. The major anatomic area of difficulty in foreign body removal is the isthmus of the external ear canal. The object is often pushed beyond the isthmus in an attempt to remove it and may come to lie against the ear drum, causing severe pain.

The initial attempt at removal should be by irrigation. The stream of the irrigation is directed superiorly to push the object out with the backwash. Some objects lend themselves to removal by a hook passed behind the object and brought forward. Unless children are very cooperative during foreign body removal it is best to use a general anesthetic to prevent injury to the tympanic membrane or ossicles during the procedure.

Infection

Inflammation of the ear canal is called external otitis, or "swimmer's ear."

EXAMINATION. The ear canal and the external ear may be red and swollen; the former may be so swollen that the tympanic membrane cannot be seen. External otitis is very painful, and the patients may be quite ill.

TREATMENT OF ACUTE LOCALIZED EXTERNAL OTITIS. If the ear canal alone is involved in the inflammation, a cotton pledget impregnated with Cortisporin ointment is inserted to fill the external ear canal. If the external ear (pinna) is also involved, the area of inflamed skin is treated with 0.5% triamcinolone ointment. Cortisporin otic drops are applied to the cotton wick four times daily. The cotton wick is removed after 48 hours, and the drops continued in the ear canal for 1 week.

External otitis with complications should be treated on an inpatient basis. Patients with severe external otitis should be checked for diabetes.

MIDDLE EAR: OTITIS MEDIA

Patients with otitis media are often toxic, with a high fever and severe pain.

Examination

Examination of the ear reveals a red, swollen, immobile tympanic membrane. Tuning fork tests reveal a conductive hearing loss (bone conduction greater than air conduction, or negative Rinne).

Treatment

GENERAL MEASURES. The treatment of acute otitis media includes the administration of antibiotics, antihistamines, nasal decongestants, and analgesics. The patient should be watched for the possible development of complications.

MYRINGOTOMY. Emergency outpatient myringotomy is indicated under the following circumstances: (1) when the tympanic membrane is red and swollen and the patient has a high fever and severe unremitting pain; (2) when it is necessary to identify the organism causing otitis media with complications, including mastoiditis and meningitis.

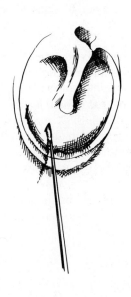

Emergency outpatient myringotomy is carried out as follows:

Local anesthesia for the ear canal is given as described under Local Anesthesia. An operating microscope is used to make certain the incision is correctly placed. The myringotomy incision is made anterior and inferior to the handle of the malleus, to protect the ossicles. Following myringotomy, the fluid or pus is suctioned and sent for culture. Myringotomy tubes are not placed in patients with acute otitis media.

SALIVARY GLANDS
Emergency problems involving the salivary glands include inflammation, stones, and foreign bodies.

Inflammation: Acute Parotitis
Inflammation of the submandibular or parotid glands with or without abscess formation may be due to blockage of the duct from inflammation or a foreign body, or to extension of infection from neighboring structures.

EXAMINATION. Parotitis is common in dehydrated elderly patients. There is pain and tenderness of the gland, especially after eating. Palpation of the gland reveals swelling, firmness, and, rarely, fluctuance. Pus may be milked from Stensen's duct. Soft tissue films of the neck may reveal the presence of a stone.

TREATMENT. The patient is given adequate hydration, antibiotics effective against gram positive-organisms, and warm saline soaks.

Elderly dehydrated patients with acute parotitis should be admitted to the hospital because of the markedly increased morbidity and mortality associated with this disease in the elderly. Incision and drainage of this area should be done on an inpatient basis.

Salivary Gland Stones

Stones may form in any of the salivary glands or their ducts, but are most often found in the submandibular gland and Wharton's duct. They are less common in the parotid gland and Stenson's duct. They are composed largely of phosphate and carbonate of calcium and are usually radiopaque.

EXAMINATION. Calculi usually produce the symptoms of duct obstruction, with secondary infection in the gland induced by stasis. Palpation of the floor of the mouth or cheek may reveal the stone. Probing of the duct with lacrimal duct probes will occasionally reveal a palpable stone.

ROENTGENOGRAMS. Soft tissue films, including an occlusal dental view, may sometimes reveal the stone. A sialogram will reveal the presence of nonopaque stones. In the figure, the orifice of Stenson's duct is identified above the upper second molar (A), and Hypaque dye is injected into the duct (B) through a plastic cannula.

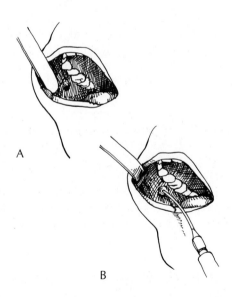

TREATMENT. The calculus may pass spontaneously. If not, dilation of the duct and probing may dislodge the stone, or surgical removal may be required.

Surgical removal of submandibular or parotid gland calculi can often be done on an outpatient basis under local anesthesia. After topical and infiltration of lidocaine over the palpable stone, an incision is made over the stone in Wharton's duct (A, B) or Stenson's duct (C, D). The stone is grasped with forceps and removed.

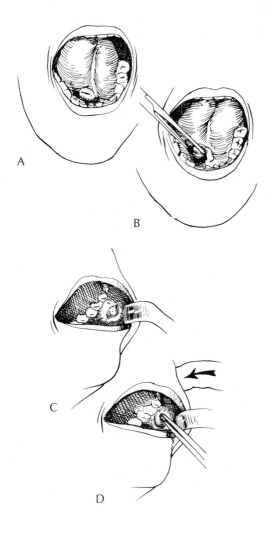

Trauma to the Parotid Duct

Trauma to the parotid duct is seldom an isolated feature in a facial injury. It should be searched for in any patient with a traumatic injury to the cheek.

TREATMENT. An isolated laceration of the parotid duct may be marsupialized by suturing the cut edges of the duct to the cut edges of the overlying mucosa using 5-0 nylon sutures to form a fistula, or reanastomosed with 5-0 nylon interrupted sutures. If the duct is reanastomosed, a polyethylene catheter is sutured in place as a stent for 2 weeks. These procedures are usually done on an inpatient basis.

Respiratory Insufficiency

Respiratory insufficiency is failure of the respiratory system to provide adequate oxygen for metabolic needs, or to remove carbon dioxide adequately from the body, or both. Causes of respiratory insufficiency include the following:

1. Depression of the respiratory center secondary to cerebral trauma, increased intracranial pressure, prolonged hypoxia, or exogenous drugs.
2. Mechanical resistance to airflow, including tumors of or trauma to the upper respiratory tract and secretional obstruction of the lower respiratory tract secondary to inflammatory disease.
3. Disturbances of the mechanical factors in respiration, including respiratory muscle paralysis, neuromuscular block, chest trauma, and emphysema and other intrinsic pulmonary diseases.

EXAMINATION

Patients with mechanical obstruction present with difficulty in breathing and exhibit inspiratory stridor. Retractions and cyanosis are often present. Tachycardia and hypotension indicate the seriousness of the situation. Examination of the upper airway, including the nose, nasopharynx, oral cavity, hypopharynx, oropharynx, and larynx, may indicate the possibility of upper airway obstruction. Neurologic examination may indicate a cause. Chest roentgenograms and blood gas determinations, including pH, Pco_2, O_2 saturation, and Po_2, are helpful.

TREATMENT

Oropharyngeal or Nasal Intubation

INDICATIONS. Airway obstruction due to trauma or lesions of the oral cavity are treated by oropharyngeal or nasal airway intubation.

TECHNIQUE. Oropharyngeal airways are placed in the mouth to bypass the oral cavity obstruction. Standard nasal airways placed through the nose into the oropharynx will bypass the oral cavity obstruction.

Endotracheal Intubation

INDICATIONS. Endotracheal intubation is the most rapid method of establishing an airway in patients with acute respiratory insufficiency. It is indicated (1) for temporary respiratory problems, (2) when tracheostomy equipment is unavailable, and (3) as a precursor to tracheostomy, particularly in infants. It provides immediate control of the airway, precluding a hasty tracheostomy.

TECHNIQUE. Topical lidocaine (1%) is used when necessary. The oral cavity and pharynx are sprayed, and cotton pledgets soaked in lidocaine are applied to the pyriform fossae using the Jackson cross-action forceps. Lidocaine is dripped onto the vocal cords or injected into the subglottic area through the cricothyroid membrane.

The patient is placed in the supine position, and the neck is extended anteriorly. The larynx is exposed with a laryngoscope, and a large endotracheal tube or a bronchoscope or catheter is inserted into the trachea. With the airway safely under control, the patient is admitted for definitive treatment (Chap. 2).

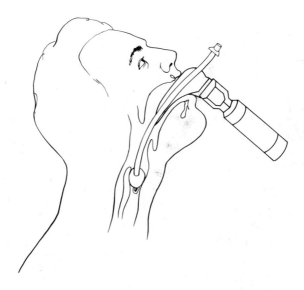

Cricothyrotomy

When endotracheal intubation is not possible, either tracheostomy or cricothyrotomy (cricoconiotomy) may be necessary for acute respiratory obstruction. Tracheostomy is the better procedure, but under certain emergency conditions, cricothyrotomy may be lifesaving.

INDICATIONS. Cricothyrotomy is performed when equipment and instruments to perform endotracheal intubation or tracheostomy are unavailable; or it may be used as a rapid standard method of establishing an airway by nonsurgically trained personnel.

TECHNIQUE. The cricothyroid space is identified by extending the patient's head and palpating the prominent arch of the cricoid cartilage below the palpable margin of the thyroid cartilage. While the area is fixed with one hand, a small horizontal incision is made with any sharp instrument (such as a penknife) just above the upper part of the cricoid cartilage. The cricothyroid membrane is punctured in the midline. The puncture wound is enlarged and a thin-walled, blunt, hollow instrument is forced into the trachea. This may be part of a ball point pen, as shown, or one or more No. 15 hypodermic needles may be inserted in extreme conditions when no other equipment is available.

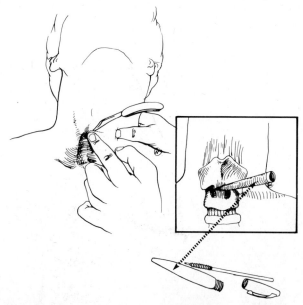

Nasotracheal Intubation

INDICATIONS. Nasotracheal intubation should be utilized when airway care for less than 48 to 72 hours is anticipated. It is particularly useful in the pediatric age group. Some of the more common indications include inflammatory diseases of the oral cavity, subglottis, larynx, trachea, and lung. Nasotracheal intubation should not be used for acute epiglottitis.

TECHNIQUE. A standard endotracheal tube is inserted through the nose into the hypopharynx and then directed through the larynx with a laryngoscope and a McGill forceps. It is then taped in place, and the patient is admitted for definitive care.

Tracheostomy

INDICATIONS. Tracheostomy should be performed when airway care for more than 48 to 72 hours is anticipated. Elective tracheostomy is performed in patients undergoing major head and neck, intracranial, or thoracic operations or in patients with chronic pulmonary insufficiency.

Therapeutic tracheostomy is performed in patients with respiratory insufficiency due to alveolar hypoventilation or secretional anoxia, or to provide for the use of mechanical artificial respiration.

TECHNIQUE. When possible, endotracheal intubation or placement of a bronchoscope should be performed prior to therapeutic tracheostomy, particularly in children. If intubation is not possible, ventilation and oxygenation using an Ambu bag and mask are valuable. Orderly tracheostomy demands previous control of the airway.

The patient should lie supine with a folded sheet under the shoulders to allow maximal extension of the neck. This may be done in the semirecumbent position. In adults, a local anesthetic is well tolerated; general anesthesia is used only if an endotracheal tube is in position. Local anesthesia is obtained by infiltrating the skin in the line of incision and depositing lidocaine in the deeper midline tissues to the level of the anterior tracheal wall.

The skin incision is determined by the circumstances. A true emergency tracheostomy in which control of the airway is not possible demands a vertical skin incision. An orderly, controlled tracheostomy allows for horizontal skin incision. Most tracheostomies in infants should be done through a vertical skin incision.

The skin incision is deepened down to the strap muscles. The strap muscles are separated vertically in the midline and retracted laterally. This exposes the pretracheal fascia, which covers the trachea and the thyroid isthmus. When possible, the tracheostomy is done either above or below the thyroid isthmus.

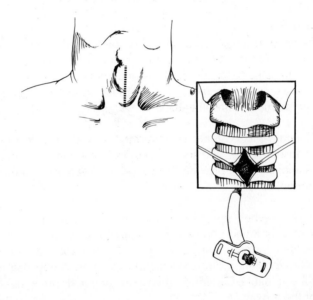

The trachea is then identified and fixed by inserting a hook in the anterior wall between the first and second ring, pulling the trachea in an upward and outward direction. The tracheal incision should not extend above the first tracheal ring. A vertical incision is made through the trachea, and cartilage is not removed. In infants and children, two individual 2-0 black silk sutures are inserted to help with identification of the tracheostomy should accidental extubation occur. The tracheal incision is spread with a large hemostat, and a tube of appropriate size is inserted immediately.

Some patients may become apneic due to loss of hypoxic respiratory drive. This should be anticipated and artificial respiration instituted if necessary. The inserted tracheostomy tube should have a low pressure cuff to allow for mechanical respiration.

The skin incision should not be sutured or dressed tightly, since this may lead to the development of subcutaneous emphysema, pneumomediastinum, and pneumothorax. A small gauze pad may be placed between the flange of the tube and the skin of the neck.

The patient is admitted to the hospital for definitive treatment of the respiratory problem. If at all possible, elective tracheostomy is performed under operating room conditions.

INFLAMMATION OF THE LARYNX
Acute inflammation of the larynx may cause severe respiratory distress and may progress to total airway obstruction and death. Of major importance is the differentiation between epiglottitis (acute supraglottic laryngitis) and croup (acute laryngotracheobronchitis). Epiglottitis is inflammation of the supraglottic structures and tends to affect children from 3 to 6 years of age, but also occurs in adults. It is a potentially lethal disease. Croup is an inflammatory process of the subglottic larynx, trachea, and bronchi involving children under the age of 5 years.

Epiglottitis
Acute epiglottitis is a severe bacterial cellulitis of the tissues of the epiglottis and aryepiglottic folds. Obstruction of the laryngeal vestibule prevents effective cough and removal of secretions, creating a secondary obstructive problem. The course of this disease may include progression from mild upper respiratory infection to almost complete respiratory obstruction over a period of 6 to 12 hours.

EXAMINATION. The voice is not usually hoarse but has a muffled quality, as though the patient had a hot potato in his mouth. Sore throat, fever, dysphagia, and pain are present. Respiratory distress with exhaustion and circulatory collapse may develop. Examination of the oral cavity with a tongue depressor may reveal a fiery-red, edemanous epiglottis that is diagnostic. Extreme caution must be used during the examination, since acute obstruction may be precipitated. Roentgenograms of the neck will indicate a characteristic supraglottic swelling encroaching on the airway.

TREATMENT. Immediate hospitalization in an intensive care unit is indicated. Nasotracheal or endotracheal intubation of these patients is extremely difficult and dangerous. Early tracheostomy is indicated in most patients. After securing a safe airway, broad-spectrum antibiotic coverage is begun.

Croup
As noted, croup is an acute inflammatory disease of the subglottic larynx, trachea, and bronchi. The usual etiologic agent is viral. There is edema in the region of the subglottic area at the conus elasticus, with resultant marked swelling of the narrowest portion of the airway.

The characteristic croupy, "barky," nonproductive cough of croup usually follows an upper respiratory tract infection. Increasing respiratory difficulty with stridor may occur. Fever, retractions, restlessness, refusal to take food, and tachycardia follow.

EXAMINATION. Acute epiglottitis must be ruled out. Roentgenograms of the neck reveal subglottic narrowing. Chest films confirm the presence or absence of concomitant pneumonia.

TREATMENT. Mild croup (without pneumonia) may be treated with humidification, hydration, oxygen, and antibiotic therapy. Solu-Cortef, 100 mg, is given intravenously in the acute phase of the disease. Response to this medication, if it occurs, should be noted in the first several hours. Positive-pressure breathing with aerosolized norepinephrine is given by mask.

If this regimen is not immediately effective in the management of the respiratory distress, the patient is admitted to the hospital. Certain hospitals have outpatient therapy units for the exclusive treatment of this disease, and croup patients are admitted directly to such units.

Nasotracheal intubation is indicated when obstruction with cyanosis, tachycardia, and a decrease in pulmonary ventilation is present. Most patients will respond to conservative measures and will not require nasotracheal intubation if therapy is instituted early enough.

After 48 to 72 hours of nasotracheal intubation the tube is removed, and the patient is observed for respiratory distress. If the stridor and respiratory problems are still present, the patient is reintubated, and an orderly elective tracheotomy is performed.

AIRWAY FOREIGN BODIES
Every patient with acute and chronic pulmonary symptoms should be suspected of having a foreign body. Of practical importance is the position of the foreign body in the airway.

Acute Airway Obstruction: Food Choking
Food choking is easily recognized. The victim cannot speak or breathe, becomes pale and cyanotic, and collapses. A universal signal has been suggested in which the victim grasps his neck between thumb and index finger of one hand to signal he is choking on food. The Heimlich procedure to prevent food choking is discussed in Chapter 1.

Peripheral Bronchial Foreign Body
EXAMINATION. In all patients with choking, coughing, and cyanosis a bronchial foreign body should be suspected. Examination of the pharynx, hypopharynx, and larynx usually reveals nothing abnormal, but auscultation of the lungs may reveal signs of air trapping.

ROENTGENOGRAMS. Roentgenograms of the chest in inspiratory and expiratory phases and cinefluorography are usually diagnostic, even if the foreign body is not radiopaque.

TREATMENT. Patients with peripheral foreign bodies with no acute respiratory distress should be admitted to the hospital for bronchoscopy and removal of the foreign body.

Foreign Bodies of the Esophagus

Patients present with the feeling of foreign body in the throat. They may also complain of being short of breath. They can usually pinpoint the type of foreign body involved and the exact position where they feel the impaction.

EXAMINATION. Thorough examination of the oral cavity, nasopharynx, and base of tongue and hypopharynx may reveal the foreign body. A mirror must be used to examine these areas adequately. Palpation is of particular importance. Roentgenograms of the cervical esophagus taken during deglutition, using a barium-impregnated cotton pledget, may reveal a nonradiopaque foreign body.

TREATMENT. Foreign bodies in the oral cavity and at the base of the tongue can usually be removed in the outpatient department. Patients with foreign bodies in the hypopharynx and the esophagus are admitted to the hospital for definitive care.

LARYNGEAL TRAUMA

Blunt trauma to the neck is usually caused by an automobile accident in which the extended neck hits the dashboard or steering wheel.

Examination

Patients with blunt trauma to the neck present with stridor, dysphonia or aphonia, cough, neck pain, dysphagia or odynophagia, increasing airway obstruction, and subcutaneous emphysema. The presence of subcutaneous emphysema and increasing airway obstruction are cardinal signs of disruption of the larynx or trachea.

Treatment

Initial treatment requires establishment of an adequate airway. Early tracheostomy is mandatory. This is followed by admission to the hospital for detailed assessment of the injury and determination of the necessity for further definitive treatment to be carried out immediately or to be delayed, whichever is dictated by the clinical situation.

PENETRATING INJURY TO THE NECK

Penetrating wounds of the neck demand immediate evaluation and management. Outpatient management only includes stabilization of the patient's condition to prepare him for admission to the hospital.

Examination

Thorough evaluation of the patient is critical. After stabilization of the patient's condition, including establishment of an airway, stopping the hemorrhage, and preparations for and replacement of blood and fluid loss, a thorough search for the following kinds of injury is important:

VASCULAR INJURY. A search is made for the site of hemorrhage, expanding hematoma, signs of compression or displacement of the trachea, bruit, absence of pulse in the extremities, and pulses in the superficial temporal, facial, or retinal arteries or central nervous system deficit. Soft tissue roentgenograms of the neck for cervical neck spaces are taken. Arteriograms are often indicated for complete evaluation.

RESPIRATORY TRACT INJURY. Signs of crepitus, dysphonia, aspiration, and hemopneumothorax are noted.

DIGESTIVE TRACT INJURY. Signs of crepitus, dysphagia, or odynophagia may be present. A barium or Hypaque-swallow roentgenogram may show extravasation of dye.

NERVOUS SYSTEM INJURY. Cranial nerves, especially IX, X, XI, and XII, may be injured. The Horner syndrome may indicate an injury along the cervical sympathetic trunk. A brachial plexus deficit may be present. Hemiplegia may indicate contralateral damage to the brain by direct injury, cervical cord injury, or interruption of the carotid system.

Early examination and recording of abnormalities of these findings will help in the definitive care and subsequent results in the hospitalized patient.

Facial Nerve Paralysis

Facial palsy is not a disease but a sign of a pathologic process involving the seventh cranial nerve. Although Bell's (idiopathic) facial palsy continues to be the most common type of facial paralysis, a specific cause for the palsy will be found in about 1 in 5 patients. Table 8-1 lists the causes of facial nerve paralysis.

Examination

Patients with traumatic facial paralysis should be admitted to the hospital for further evaluation and treatment. In patients with nontraumatic facial palsy, an attempt should be made to determine the possible cause. Specific topographic diagnostic studies for facial nerve paralysis location include a general physical and complete ear, nose, and throat examinations, audiometric and vestibular examinations, roentgenograms of the mastoid and internal auditory canals, a Schirmer test for tearing, electrogustometry, tests for salivary flow, and special audiometry tests including tympanometry and stapedial reflex tests. These tests can all be performed as outpatient procedures by the specialist.

Management

The management of facial palsy is determined by the findings of the diagnostic workup.

Table 8-1. Causes of Facial Nerve Paralysis

Traumatic
    Intracranial: transection in neurosurgical procedures within cerebellopontine angle
    Intratemporal
        Surgical division in surgery of parotid gland or face
        Fracture of temporal bone
    Extratemporal
        Surgical division in surgery of parotid gland or face
        Laceration of face
Atraumatic
    Noninfectious
        Bell's palsy
        Melkersson syndrome
        Tumors of cerebellopontine angle or facial nerve
    Infectious
        Otitis media
        Herpes zoster oticus

9

Chest Procedures

John P. Connors

Significant thoracic injuries occur in almost 50 percent of those who die following automobile accidents. In most cases the physical findings are usually adequate to initiate the appropriate therapy, especially in severely traumatized patients. Life-threatening cardiac tamponade or tension pneumothorax often requires management prior to chest x-ray examination. However, a chest roentgenogram should be obtained as soon as possible, preferably with the patient in the upright position.

Examination of the Thoracic Wall
The initial examination of the patient should include the following:

1. Location and type of wounds.
2. Deformity of the chest wall.
3. Observation of respiratory efforts, including excursion of the suprasternal, supraclavicular and intercostal spaces.
4. Identification of paradoxical chest-wall motion indicating a flail segment.
5. Subcutaneous emphysema.
6. Distention of the neck veins.
7. The effectiveness of the patient's ventilation indicated by the color of the nail beds and lips.

If a sucking wound or an open wound is present, an airtight seal must be obtained by covering the area with a plastic film or grease gauze dressing. The latter is reinforced with a dry gauze pad and adhesive tape until definitive wound care can be provided.

Rib Fracture
Fractured ribs may be very painful, thereby limiting adequate ventilation and coughing. To control the pain, an intercostal block is performed using 1% lidocaine anesthesia. Infiltration of two interspaces above and two below the involved ribs ensures more complete analgesia (Chap. 5). Adhesive strapping is not advised, since restricting ventilation may promote infection of the lung.

Flail Chest

Paradoxical chest wall motion following extensive injury may result in severe hypoventilation, the management of which requires endotracheal intubation or tracheostomy and assisted ventilation. Sudden deterioration in the patient's condition while on the ventilator may be a result of the development of a tension pneumothorax, requiring urgent chest tube insertion.

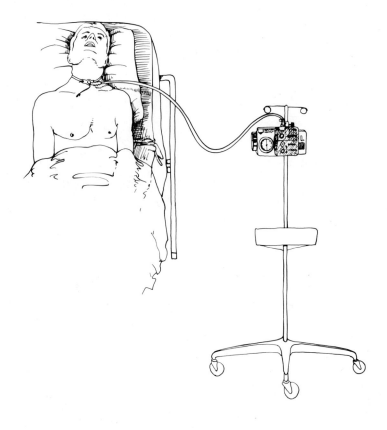

If a ventilator is not available, paradoxical respirations and hypoventilation may be controlled by stabilizing the flail segment with a large towel clip. Traction with a 2-pound weight is maintained, and repeated intercostal blocks for analgesia are carried out.

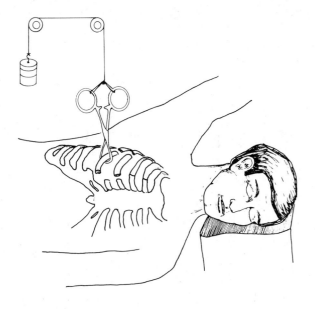

Thoracentesis
Traumatic hemothorax or pneumothorax is best managed by chest tube insertion. Thoracentesis should be reserved for the treatment of small bloody or pleural fluid collections. A large-gauge needle is inserted in the appropriate lower interspace in the posterior axillary line (A). The intercostal neurovascular bundle is avoided by penetrating the pleural space immediately above the underlying rib. The needle is held at the proper insertion depth by applying a clamp where it pierces the skin (B).

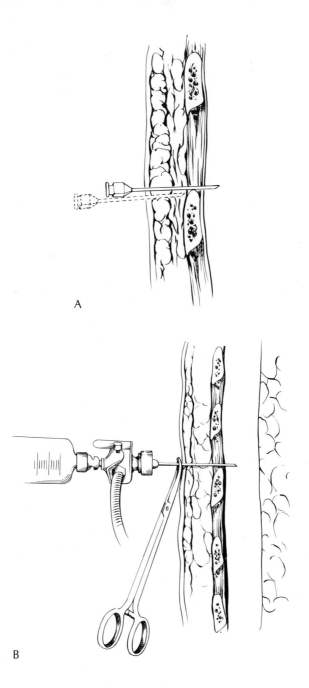

A

B

Chest Tube Insertion

The ideal point of insertion for a chest tube in a traumatic hemothorax or pneumothorax is located a handbreadth below the axilla in the midaxillary line.

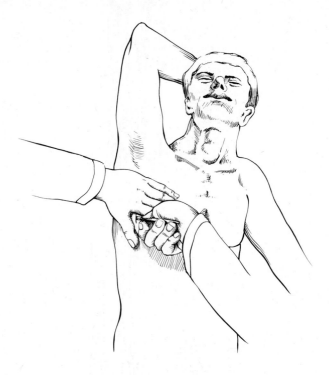

An anterior point for chest tube insertion may be considered when the chest roentgenogram indicates the presence of a pneumothorax only. Sterile preparation and isolation of the field with towels is carried out, and a small area over the second interspace in the midclavicular line is infiltrated with 1% lidocaine anesthesia. A transverse short (1-inch) skin incision is then made.

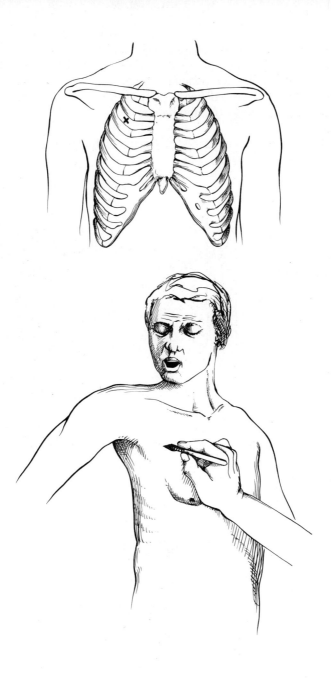

The chest tube may be inserted with or without a trocar. In the latter case, blunt dissection with a clamp is used to spread the intercostal muscles and penetrate the pleura. After the chest has been opened, a gloved finger must be inserted to palpate the space and determine that the lung is free.

A No. 28 tube is then grasped at the end with a Kelly clamp and inserted into the pleural space.

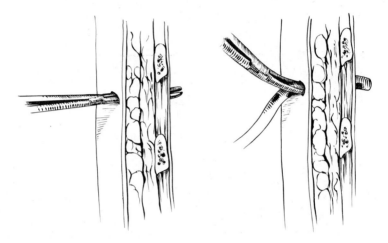

The tube is advanced until the last hole is well within the thoracic cavity. It is then fixed to the chest wall with a heavy silk or nylon suture.

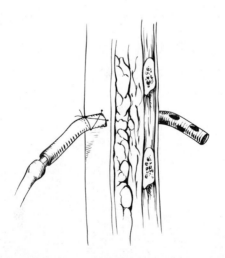

Trocar Insertion of a Chest Tube

If a trocar is available, the chest wall preparation and incision are similar. Controlled and firm rotation of the trocar is performed until penetration of the pleural space is achieved. The central obturator is removed and a clamped chest tube inserted. The sleeve is removed, leaving the clamped chest tube in place.

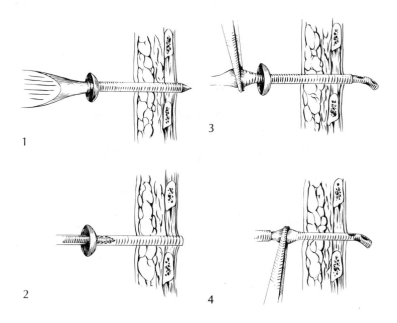

1

2

3

4

The chest tube remains clamped until it is connected to water-seal drainage. The end of the chest tube should be no more than 4 cm below the fluid level in the water-seal bottle to allow complete drainage of fluid and air from the chest.

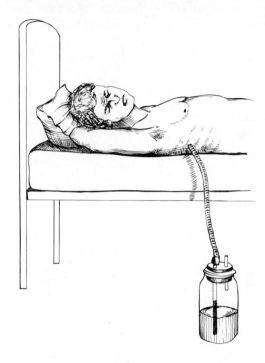

To avoid the problem of excessive fluid accumulation, a collecting bottle may be interposed in the drainage system.

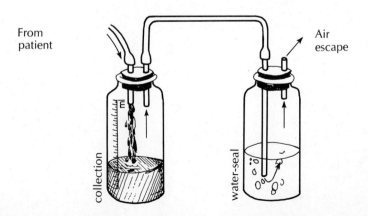

From patient

Air escape

collection

water-seal

Connecting the system to a vacuum pump will speed the reexpansion of the lung and evacuation of fluid. The interposition of a third bottle to regulate the level of negative suction pressure at 25 cm of water is recommended. Self-enclosed and sterile commercial versions of triple bottle systems are available.

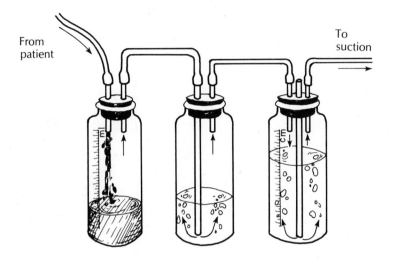

From
patient

To
suction

Autotransfusion

Autotransfusion of blood lost in the intrapleural space should be considered as a means of resuscitating patients in profound shock. The uncontaminated blood may be collected in a sterile bottle partially filled with saline. Before reinfusion, the blood must be filtered to eliminate small clots and other particulate matter.

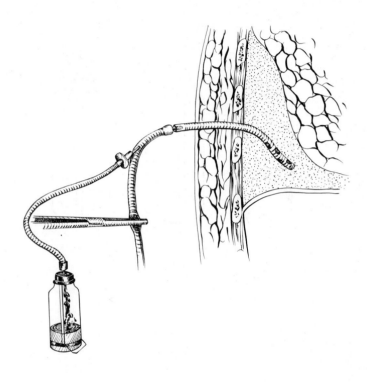

Chest Valves for Pneumothorax

A severe tension pneumothorax must be immediately relieved either by: (1) the temporary insertion of a large-bore needle into the chest cavity, or (2) slitting the end of a condom or finger cot and tying it over the needle hub, creating a one-way valve mechanism.

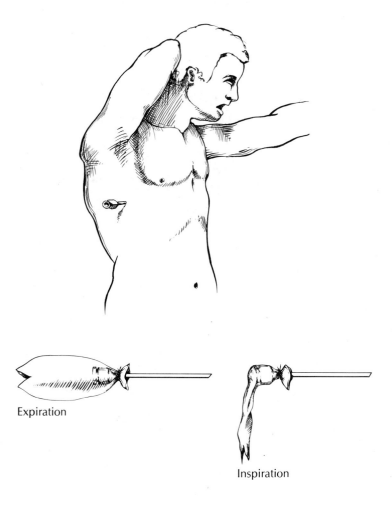

Expiration

Inspiration

Pericardiocentesis

The diagnosis of pericardial tamponade is made by observing:

1. Distended veins in the neck.
2. A low blood pressure.
3. Tachycardia and diminished or absent heart sounds.
4. Elevated venous pressure.

The head of the stretcher or bed is elevated 60°. After skin preparation, a 16-gauge, short bevel needle, connected to a 50-ml syringe is inserted to the left of the xiphoid cartilage at a 45° angle to the skin. It is advanced toward the right shoulder with suction applied until unclotted blood is aspirated.

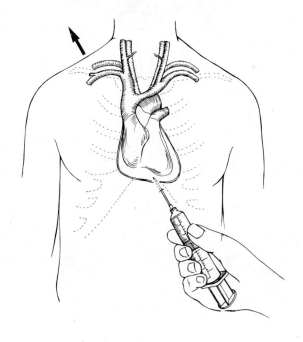

A complication of pericardiocentesis is penetration of the inferior surface of the heart, which may be avoided by connecting the aspirating needle to the chest lead of an electrocardiograph with sterile alligator clamps and wire. An electrocardiograph tracing made from this lead will demonstrate a normal pattern; however, elevation of the S–T segment of the tracing or extrasystoles indicates that the wall of the ventricle is being touched.

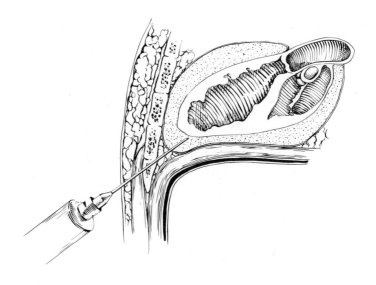

10

Abdominal Techniques

Allen P. Klippel

Regional Anatomy

In considering abdominal problems, a careful history of the onset of the disease or how the injury was suffered, coupled with a careful, meticulous examination of the abdominal areas, will almost always make the diagnosis apparent. Diagnostic techniques can never replace the eye, ear, and gentle fingers of the skilled physician, and laboratory and roentgenographic tests must be of secondary interest. History taking is of paramount importance in making the diagnosis of a disease process; even in the traumatized patient, it is essential to know how the injuring force was applied, in what condition the patient was found, and how he reacted during the period before arrival at the hospital.

In considering the abdominal cavity, it is necessary to define the regions in an accepted manner and to remember the organs normally located in each region.

The abdomen is arbitrarily divided into four quadrants by perpendicular lines drawn through the umbilicus.

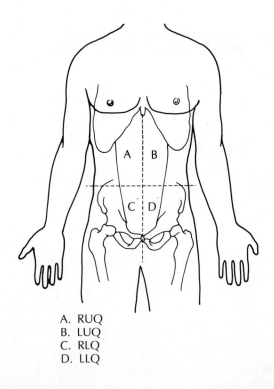

A. RUQ
B. LUQ
C. RLQ
D. LLQ

In addition, certain other areas are frequently delineated, namely, the epigastric, central abdomen or periumbilical, supra-pubic, right and left hypochondria, and right and left iliac or inguinal areas.

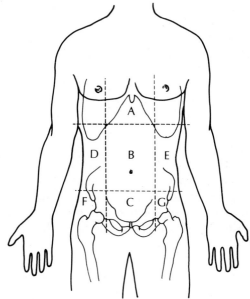

A. Epigastric
B. Central Abdomen
C. Suprapubic
D. R. Hypochondrium
E. L. Hypochondrium
F. R. Iliac
G. L. Iliac

The quadrants and areas, and their contents, are as follows:

1. Right upper quadrant (RUQ): Liver, gallbladder, hepatic flex-ure of the colon, right kidney.
2. Left upper quadrant (LUQ): Spleen, splenic flexure of colon, left kidney, tail of the pancreas.
3. Epigastrium: Stomach and duodenum, left lobe of liver, head and body of the pancreas, transverse colon.
4. Right lower quadrant (RLQ): Cecum, appendix and ascending colon, distal small bowel, right uterine tube and ovary.
5. Left lower quadrant (LLQ): Descending and sigmoid colon, left uterine tube and ovary.
6. Umbilical area: Small intestine and possibly transverse colon.
7. Suprapubic: Urinary bladder, female genital organs.

Examination

INSPECTION

Inspection of the surface of the abdomen is first done to note the following:

1. Presence of scars.
2. Contour, including abnormal protrusions.
3. Presence of dilated veins.
4. Visible peristalsis.
5. Abdominal-wall movement coupled with respirations.
6. Condition of the umbilical area, e.g., protrusion or discoloration.

PALPATION

The table or bed on which the patient is lying must be high enough so that the hand of the examining physician does not have to be hyperextended at the wrist. By putting a pillow under the patient's knees, or by putting the patient's feet flat on the table after bending the knees the patient will be encouraged to relax the abdominal musculature.

The palpating hand and fingers should be held parallel to the abdomen. Note the presence or absence of involuntary guarding of the abdominal muscles. Downward movement of the liver or spleen with respiration will allow the edge of these organs to be palpated. The kidneys may be palpable in a thin person. Examine the area of possible disease only after the rest of the abdomen has been palpated.

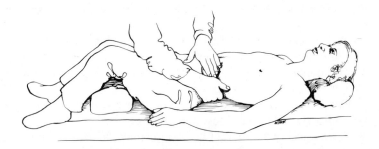

PERCUSSION

Gentle percussion can distinguish the hollow from the solid viscera. The liver can be mapped out, as can an enlarged spleen, by a
dull, percussive note as compared to the tympanitic note elicited
from the contents of the rest of the abdomen. A distended urinary
or gallbladder may similarly be detected.

Gentle percussion is especially useful in differentiating between
an acutely distended gallbladder and an inflamed appendix.
With percussion, the patient is better able to pinpoint the area of
maximal tenderness.

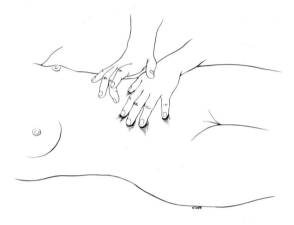

Dullness to percussion that moves as the patient is rolled from side to side indicates ascites. Transmission of an impulse across the abdomen also indicates the presence of intraabdominal fluid.

With the side of an assistant's hand compressing the fat in the midline so that a fat wave can be differentiated from a fluid wave, the examiner taps one side of the abdomen. The fingertips of the opposite hand can perceive the transmission of the tap.

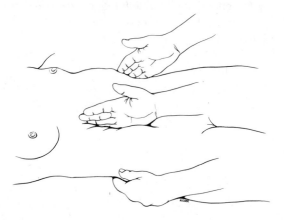

REBOUND TENDERNESS

Rebound tenderness is a sign of peritoneal irritation. Local rebound tenderness is demonstrated by gently pushing at the area of maximal tenderness, as indicated by the patient. Peritonitis must be considered if the sudden movement of the abdominal wall resulting from removing the fingers is painful at the suspected point.

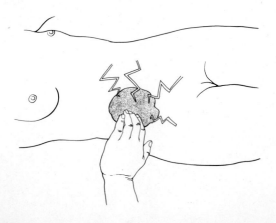

Referred rebound tenderness is elicited by pushing on the abdominal wall with the fingertips in a nontender area away from the point of pain and tenderness, then suddenly releasing the pressure. This sign is positive if the sudden movement of the abdominal wall produces pain in the suspected area.

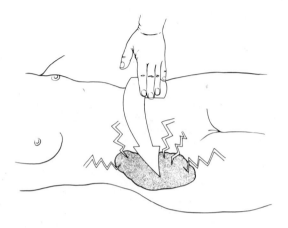

AUSCULTATION

Peristaltic activity is audible in the abdomen of most normal persons. Increased sounds with painful rushes and periods of silence may indicate intestinal obstruction. No sounds (silent abdomen for several minutes) is a common finding that accompanies peritoneal irritation. A bruit is heard over major abdominal arteries with altered intravascular flow, such as occurs with aneurysms or partial occlusions of the aorta.

HERNIAS

A hernia is indicated by an abnormal swelling, most commonly found in the epigastric, umbilical, inguinal, and femoral areas. A hernia may also be found in a scar from a prior operative procedure.

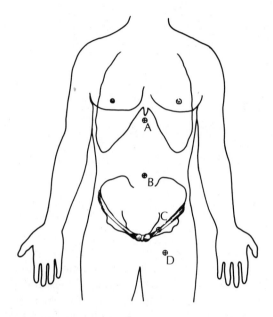

A. Epigastric
B. Umbilical
C. Inguinal
D. Femoral

Nasogastric Intubation

INDICATIONS

Intubation by a nasogastric tube should be performed when it can be reasonably expected that the stomach may be or will become distended with air or gastric secretions. The patient should be in a semisitting position if possible. Comatose patients should have an endotracheal tube inserted prior to gastric lavage to prevent gastric contents from entering the trachea.

The nasogastric tube (No. 16F for adults and No. 12F for children) may be chilled in ice. It should be well lubricated. The tube is inserted through the side of the nose with the wider aperture (check deviation of the nasal septum).

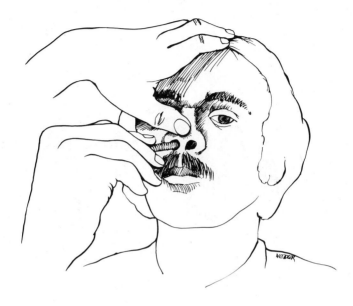

SHORT TUBES

The tube is inserted flat along the floor of the nose, not pointed upward, where it would impinge on the turbinates.

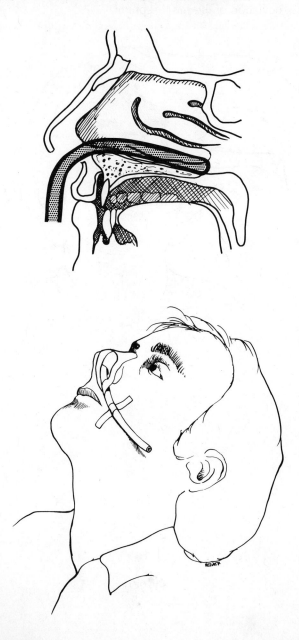

After the tube is in the posterior pharynx, the patient may aid in the passage of the tube by being instructed to hold a sip of water in his mouth, then to swallow while the tube is passed down the esophagus. If the patient coughs or becomes dyspneic, withdraw the tube to the posterior pharynx and repeat the procedure. Coughing indicates the tube was or is in the trachea.

When the tube is properly in the stomach, aspiration will produce gastric contents. Confirmation that the tube is in the stomach can be obtained by injecting 20 cc of air and listening with a stethoscope to the rumble this produces in the LUQ of the abdomen.

The tube must be taped to the nose in such a fashion that it does not produce pressure against the nares.

LONG TUBES
At the present time, passage of long tubes (Cantor or Miller-Abbott) is seldom done for intestinal obstruction except when the obstruction develops in a patient less than 4 weeks following an operation.

The tube, with the bag at the tip empty, is heavily lubricated and inserted into the nares and passed along the floor of the nasal cavity.

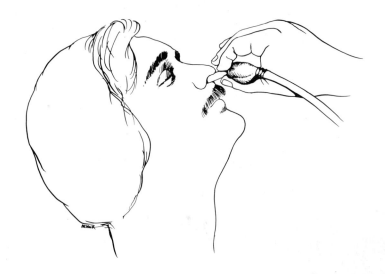

After the insertion through the nose, the tube is delivered through the mouth, and 1 ml of liquid mercury is inserted into the balloon with a syringe, using a No. 25 needle.

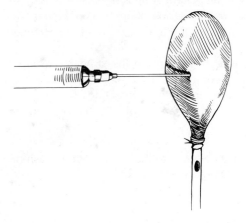

The patient is then sat upright, the mercury-filled bag is placed in the posterior pharynx, and the patient is given water to swallow. The mercury-filled bag and tube are thereby rapidly carried into the stomach.

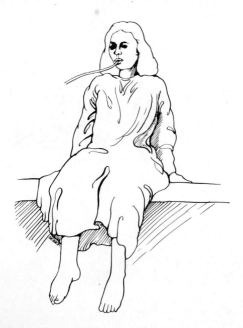

After passage, the tube is usually manipulated into or to the pylorus under fluoroscopic observation by a radiologist. This is aided by having the patient lie on the right side.

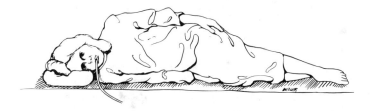

After the pylorus has been passed, as determined by the radiologist, the tube is connected to a suction machine. The tube should continue to pass down the intestine by itself and should never be taped to the nose. The tube should advance about 2.5 to 5.0 cm per hour. Initially, the patient may lie on the left side, but once the tube starts to advance, should lie supine.

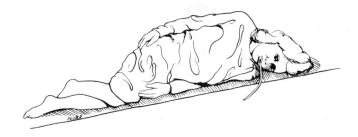

To remove a long tube when the obstruction has been relieved, pull out about 10 cm and tape to the face. Repeat this process of extracting 10 cm per hour until the tube is in the stomach, at which time it is quickly removed.

SENGSTAKEN-BLAKEMORE TUBE

The Sengstaken-Blakemore tube is a triple-lumen tube that is used to control massive bleeding from esophageal varices. It is used only in an emergency, to prepare the patient for an elective portosystemic shunt.

Spray the nose and the posterior pharynx with a local anesthetic solution. Check the balloons for leaks and lubricate the tube well. The tube is passed through the nose, using the less obstructed side. The tube should be inserted to the 50-cm mark. When the stomach has been reached, gastric contents admixed with blood should be obtained. Instill 20 cc of air and auscultate over the LUQ to confirm that the tube is in the proper position.

Inflate the gastric balloon with 50 cc of air and retract the tube until resistance is met, which indicates that the balloon is lodged at the esophagogastric junction.

Fit a football helmet with a face guard on the patient. Tape the tube to the face guard, straight out from the nose. This avoids pressure on the nose that could produce necrosis of the skin or nasal cartilages. The stomach is lavaged with copious amounts of iced saline until the return is clear.

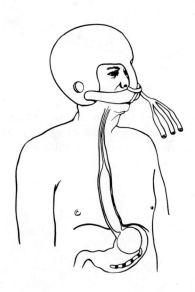

If bleeding continues, the esophageal balloon may be inflated to a pressure of 40 mm Hg. The stomach is again lavaged with iced saline until clear. After the esophageal balloon is inflated, a small nasogastric tube is inserted through the opposite nares to check for bleeding and to remove saliva. The esophageal balloon should be deflated after 24 hours. If bleeding persists with the esophageal balloon inflated, another source of hemorrhage must be suspected.

Aspiration of Peritoneal Cavity

Insertion of a needle or a tube through the abdominal wall is usually done as a diagnostic aid in certain exceptional cases. A peritoneal tap cannot replace a careful examination and should be done only when laparotomy is *not* contemplated. Before aspiration or lavage, the bladder must be empty.

INDICATIONS

Suspected Intraabdominal Hemorrhage
from a Ruptured Viscus
Taps have their greatest value when the patient is unconscious or is not cognizant of his abdomen because of spinal cord damage or another neurologic deficit.

Acute Pancreatitis
If nontraumatic pancreatitis is suspected and laparotomy is to be avoided, aspiration of the peritoneal fluid on which an amylase determination can be made will aid in confirming the diagnosis. The amylase content of the fluid aspirated must be over 100 Somogyi units per deciliter.

Suspected Intraabdominal Malignancy
In suspected intraabdominal malignant disease, any fluid that can be aspirated is submitted for cell studies, and a laparotomy may be avoided if malignant cells are found.

FOUR-QUADRANT TAP

The abdomen is shaved and prepared with soap and water, then painted with a germicide. If the patient is conscious, a local anesthetic is infiltrated at each of the four sites. The sites must be lateral to the rectus sheath to avoid hitting the epigastric blood vessels. *Do not attempt any aspirations through or near operative scars;* the intestine may be adherent at these areas.

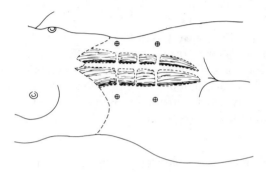

Aspiration is performed using a 1½-inch 21-gauge needle on a 10-ml syringe. If the abdomen is very obese, a 21-gauge spinal needle may be used. *Do not attempt aspiration if the abdomen is tympanitic and distended, indicating obstruction.* The normal collapsed intestine is hard to penetrate and, if stuck, will not leak. But distended intestine will leak fecal matter into the peritoneal cavity if penetrated by the needle. The tap is positive for intraabdominal hemorrhage if the blood that is removed exceeds 2 ml and *does not clot.*

If the fluid that is removed is not bloody, it should be checked for amylase or bile. Bile-stained fluid is indicative of a ruptured duodenum or gallbladder. Serous fluid should also be submitted for culture after a Gram stain of the smear has been made.

Peritoneal Dialysis
INDICATIONS
Peritoneal dialysis is indicated under the following circumstances:

1. When there are no hemodialysis facilities for a patient in renal shutdown with a toxic blood level of potassium. In an emergency, peritoneal dialysis may be done in almost any hospital, regardless of size.
2. When vascular access in a patient with a short-term problem is limited.
3. When there is transient deterioration in a patient with a chronic renal problem who is not yet a candidate for hemodialysis.
4. When a patient has severe hypotension, precluding hemodialysis.
5. In initial management of chronic renal failure, awaiting maturation of a new arteriovenous fistula.

PREOPERATIVE ROUTINE

1. The patient must fast for 12 hours before the procedure.
2. Fluids by mouth are restricted for 12 hours before the procedure.
3. Shave the skin widely around the umbilicus and adjacent abdomen.
4. Have the patient void before the procedure.
5. Sedation may be provided by administering 5 to 10 mg of diazapam intravenously or intramuscularly at the start of the procedure.

INSERTION OF PERITONEAL DIALYSIS CATHETER
Make sure the patient's bladder is empty before starting the procedure.

The usual site for the catheter to be inserted is 2 to 3 cm below the umbilicus in the midline. After the site has been prepared, it is infiltrated with lidocaine.

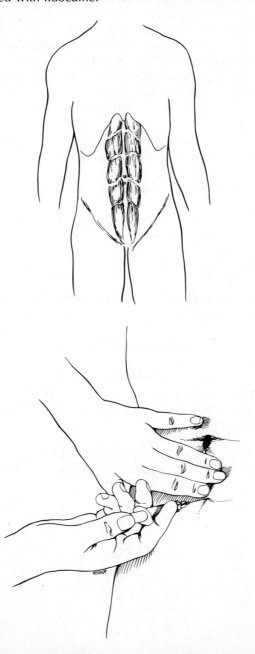

A 0.5-cm incision is made through the skin and fascia with a No. 11 blade. All abdominal scars must be avoided in selecting a site for the catheter; the bowel may be adherent to such scars and may be damaged by the catheter and trochar. If the patient has a midline scar, make the incision lateral to the rectus muscle, on the right side. Some physicians prefer to fill the abdomen with 1,000 ml of the dialysate solution through a No. 21 intravenous needle prior to inserting the catheter.

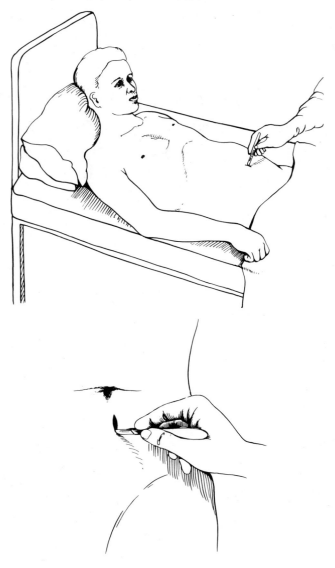

Plastic catheters designed for intravenous fluids should not be used, since they have only one hole and may become plugged. The dialysis catheter is passed through the abdominal wall while the patient raises his head to tense the muscles.

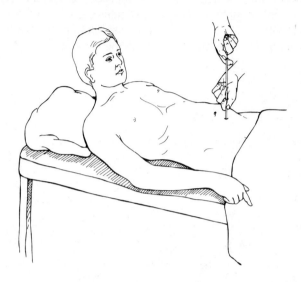

Passage through the fascia and peritoneum is signaled when the resistance to the trochar suddenly disappears.

After the peritoneum is passed, the stylette is removed.

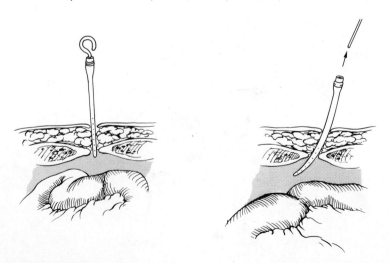

Before advancing the catheter, connect a bottle of 1,000 ml of the dialysate and start the infusion if the abdomen was not previously filled with the solution. The catheter is advanced slowly and gently to avoid injuring the bowel or bladder. The fluids are kept running as the catheter is advanced into the RLQ of the abdomen and into the right pelvic gutter.

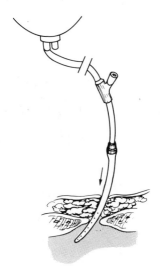

The dialysis catheter is secured to the skin with a purse-string suture of 4-0 silk. Only about 2 cm of the catheter should protrude

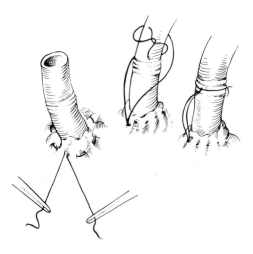

The catheter is connected to an angled adapter that must be taped to the skin. Tape should be applied to the joint between the catheter and the tubing to prevent the connection from being opened accidentally.

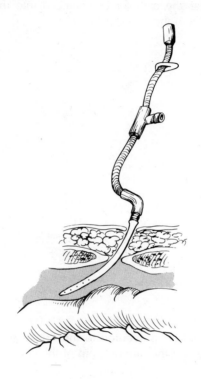

The outflow tubing is connected to a sterile urinary drainage collecting bag with a one-way valve to prevent any accidental reflux of the fluid into the abdominal cavity.

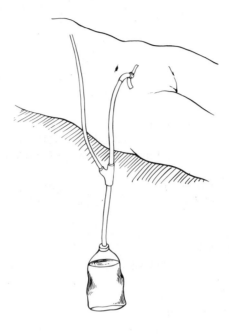

The initial lavage fluid is allowed to run into the abdomen and then is evacuated while the physician observes the first cycle to ensure that the system is functioning properly. Evacuation should occur when the bottle or bag is placed lower than the level of the patient's body. Subsequently, 1 liter of the dialysis fluid should be introduced into the peritoneal cavity over 10 minutes. The tubes are clamped for 15 minutes while equilibration occurs. The peritoneal cavity is then allowed to evacuate for 10 minutes. This cycle is repeated continuously.

Dialysis should be continued for 48 hours only. The risk of infection rises rapidly if the procedure is continued after this length of time. A physician should remove the catheter.

The composition of dialysis fluid for renal failure is as follows:

Component	Glucose 4.25% (mEq)	Glucose 1.5% (mEq)
Sodium	132	141
Calcium	3.5	3.5
Magnesium	1.5	1.5
Chloride	102	102
Sodium lactate	35	45

The osmolality of 4.25% glucose, the usual solution used, is 486 mOsm. In certain circumstances, other substances may be added to the solution. These solutions are now commercially available.

To prevent hypoalbuminemia, albumin, 3 gm per liter, should be added to the dialysis fluids used in the second 24 hours of the procedure.

COMPLICATIONS
The complications of dialysis include the following:

1. Chemical peritonitis.
2. Hypoalbuminemia.
3. Pulmonary edema.
4. Hyperglycemia. This occurs primarily in diabetic patients, but is also common in septic patients. Try to hold the blood sugar between 300 to 400 mg per deciliter. Use insulin if necessary when the blood sugar exceeds 500 mg per deciliter.
5. Hypernatremia.
6. Hypovolemia.
7. Alkalosis. (Bicarbonate ion is the least permeable.)
8. Bacterial peritonitis. This indicates that a break has occurred in sterile technique. Infection is also more likely to occur if there are leaks around the catheter site in the skin.
9. Hemorrhage. A pink color may be present in the returning dialysis fluid but this should clear with the first exchange. If bleeding persists, another, deeper stitch in the skin around the catheter may control the bleeding.
10. Perforation of a viscus. This is a remote possibility if care is taken to avoid scars and if special care is taken in advancing the catheter.

Peritoneal Lavage
The indications, hazards, and results from peritoneal lavage are approximately the same as for the four-quadrant tap. Lavage of the peritoneal cavity is, however, considerably more reliable in detecting intraabdominal hemorrhage. The technique is approximately the same as was described for dialysis. A peritoneal dialysis catheter and trochar are passed through the wall as previously described. When the fascia is penetrated, the trochar is removed and the catheter is connected to a container of 1,000 ml of Ringer's lactate. Do not use saline solution, since the pH of this solution is acid and it may induce some peritoneal irritation, possibly confusing the clinical picture. The catheter with the solution running is advanced into the right pelvic gutter. When the fluid has completely infused, the bag or bottle is placed on the floor, and the fluid is collected as it returns from the abdomen.

The tap is considered as positive for hemorrhage and indicating the need for laparotomy only when the returning fluid is so bloody that newspaper print cannot be read through the plastic intravenous tubing (approximately 100,000 red blood cells per milliliter).

Paracentesis
Paracentesis is usually performed to relieve the respiratory problems produced by distention of the abdomen with elevation of the diaphragm. The procedure will only temporarily relieve the respiratory symptoms, since the ascites usually recurs quickly. If the procedure is done to relieve a malignant effusion, one should consider the instillation of nitrogen mustard or another agent to slow the formation of fluid when the aspiration has been completed.

TECHNIQUES

All the equipment needed for the procedure is customarily wrapped on a sterile tray.

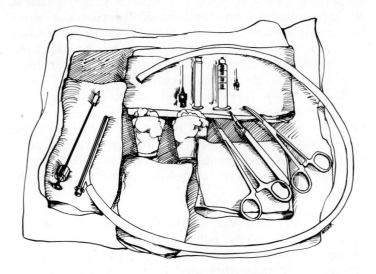

The abdomen is shaved and prepared with a germicide. The urinary bladder should be empty. The patient may sit on a chair or on the side of the bed with the feet on a chair or stool. The paracentesis point is midway between the umbilicus and pubis in the midline. A local anesthetic is introduced at this point.

The skin is incised using a No. 11 blade. The trochar with its sleeve is introduced at this point. When the peritoneum has been passed, a "give" will be felt. Remove the trochar and allow the fluid to drain. A clamp may be used to steady the tube against the abdominal wall.

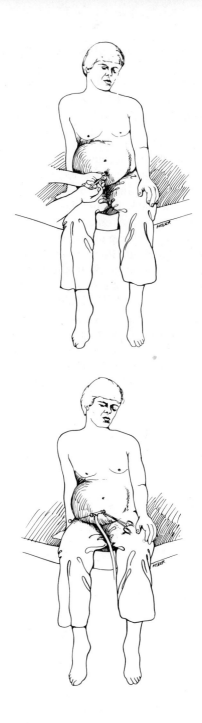

It is not advisable to remove more than 1,000 to 1,500 ml of abdominal fluid. The sudden decompression may produce syncope in some patients. When the abdominal paracentesis has been completed, a silk suture may be inserted to close the opening.

PARACENTESIS WITH REINFUSION

Ascites fluid accumulating because of hepatic failure or rupture of the cisterna chyli may be collected into a sterile collecting system and reinfused into the venous system of the patient. With the patient flat on the back, the trochar is inserted into the flank after the skin has been prepared and anesthetized. The incision should be in an area of shifting dullness. The collecting system is connected so that the ascitic fluid collects in the reinfusion bottle. An intravenous infusion of 5% dextrose in Ringer's lactate is started in a vein of the arm of the same side of the body. When the reservoir bag has been filled, it is elevated after the stopcocks are adjusted, so that the ascites fluid drains into the patient's vein. *This must not be done with a malignant effusion.* The reinfusion process is terminated when no more fluid collects in the system. The infusion rate must be monitored closely to avoid volume overload in congestive heart failure.

Pneumoperitoneum

INDICATIONS

Pneumoperitoneum is used (1) for diagnosis, i.e., to outline the viscera; (2) therapeutically, in tubercular peritonitis; and (3) to stretch the abdominal wall prior to repairing large incisional or inguinal hernias where the intestinal "right of domain" may be in question. By this mechanism the respiratory insufficiency that might follow the herniorrhaphy can be avoided. The pneumoperitoneum may be performed as an outpatient procedure, and the patient then needs to be admitted only for the operation.

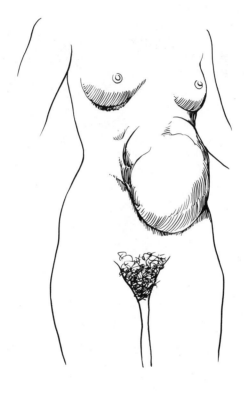

TECHNIQUES

The patient fasts for several hours. The skin around the hernia is shaved and painted with tincture of benzoin compound to protect the skin from the adhesive tape. The hernia is reduced as much as possible, and adhesive strapping is applied to keep it reduced.

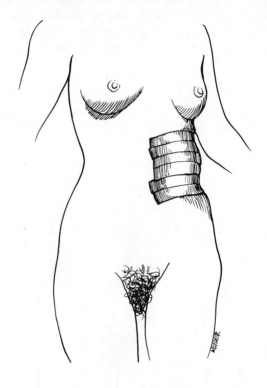

With the patient in slight Trendelenburg position, the puncture site is prepared by shaving the area and then applying a germicidal solution. The needle may be inserted in the midline of the lower abdomen, 3 cm distal to the umbilicus. Another site that may be used is midway between the anterior superior spine and either the iliac crest or the umbilicus.

The site is infiltrated with a local anesthetic, and a spinal needle is advanced into the abdomen. As the needle passes through the peritoneum, a sudden loss of resistance to the needle is felt; 10 cc of air is injected by syringe, and if it enters easily, it is almost certain that the needle is in the abdominal cavity. It is helpful to stabilize the needle with a Kelly clamp to prevent its wiggling, which could lacerate the bowel or penetrate too deeply.

Using a 100-cc syringe and a three-way stopcock, air is injected until the patient complains of discomfort, especially dyspnea. Usually, 500 to 1,000 cc can be injected at the initial session.

The patient is kept in bed for several hours and then is allowed out of bed, wearing an abdominal binder. He may then go home to return for the subsequent injections of air.

This procedure is repeated every 5 days, increasing the amount of air injected each time until as much as 6,000 to 8,000 cc of air is tolerated. Vital capacity studies should be done before and after each injection. Some reduction is anticipated after the first injection, but vital capacity should return to the preinjection value even after the subsequent injections.

The patient is considered ready to be admitted for repair when the hernia can be easily reduced, and the undistended abdominal wall is flaccid.

As larger amounts of air are required, it will be easier to inflate by the two-bottle technique: An empty sterile 1-liter intravenous bottle is connected to the abdominal needle by sterile intravenous tubing. This bottle is placed on the floor. Then a flask of 1 liter of sterile water is connected to the first bottle and allowed to run into the first bottle, thereby displacing air into the abdomen. While the tube is clamped, the bottles are reversed. The tube is then unclamped to continue the insufflation.

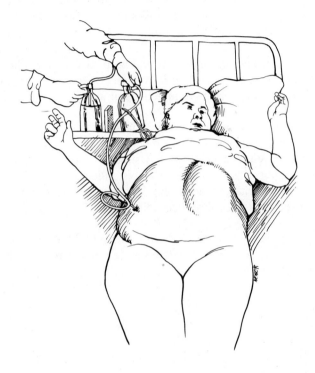

Abdominal-Wall Sinograms

Abdominal-wall sinograms are of limited value in deciding if a stab wound has penetrated the peritoneal cavity; clinical signs and symptoms are much more reliable.

The wound area is shaved and prepared, and the wound itself irrigated. It is then infiltrated with a local anesthetic. A sterile 5-ml No. 18 Foley catheter is inserted until the balloon of the catheter is in the sub Q space. A purse-string suture is tied around the catheter proximal to the balloon. The catheter balloon is inflated and then pulled back snugly against the suture.

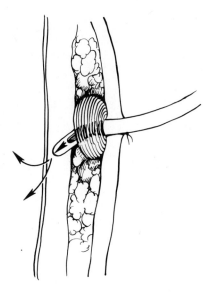

Ten ml of water-soluble radiopaque solution is then injected and roentgenograms are made of the area to see if the solution has entered the abdominal cavity.

11

Outpatient Urologic Procedures

James G. Bucy

Much of the practice of urology consists of minor operative procedures that may either be therapeutic or reparative. With the increasing concern for proper utilization of hospital beds and the rising cost of space and materials, the popularity of outpatient surgery is growing. Outpatient surgicenters are becoming increasingly prevalent and partially provide a satisfactory answer to these problems. Many urologists and surgeons are prepared to perform minor operative procedures in such facilities, or in their own offices, or in emergency departments. This chapter describes some of the urologic procedures that can or should be done on an outpatient basis.

Obviously, the situation or the patient's condition may not always allow for comfortable, convenient outpatient surgery. The decision must be based on the circumstances in the individual case. If gross contamination is present or the medical circumstances are complicated some minor procedures should not be performed in an office or emergency department setting. On the other hand, some more extensive operations, adult circumcisions, removal of foreign bodies, or debridement can be safely accomplished without hospitalization.

For the moderate number of procedures associated with some contaminated or potentially infected tissues, such as significant lacerations or "old" injuries, scrupulous preparation and topical or parenteral antibiosis is warranted.

It is particularly important that a good patient-physician relationship be established so that actual problems or fears of postoperative complications can be handled smoothly. Many problems can be avoided by frank discussion of the discomforts and risks involved. Adequate infiltrative anesthesia and gentle tissue handling promote confidence and the patient's sense of well-being. Should brief sedation be indicated, intravenous diazepam (Valium), 10 mg, can be very helpful. It must be injected slowly and the patient's status monitored carefully.

CATHETERIZATION
Types of Catheters
The types of catheters shown include the Foley (A), coudé tip
Foley (B), whistle tip (C), filiform (D), following catheter (E),
three-way catheter (for irrigation) (F).

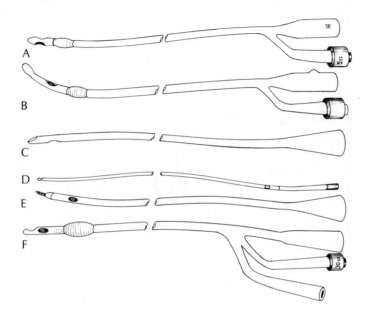

Catheterization Tray

The catheterization tray should include a 10-ml syringe (A), drapes and underpad (B), catheter (C), sterile lubricant (D), sterile disposable gloves (E), cotton balls, Septisol, and Betadine (F).

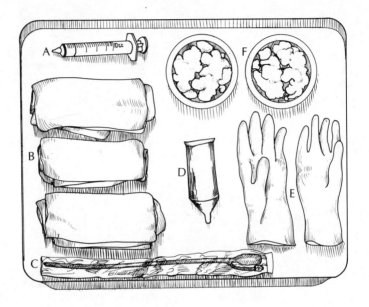

Male Catheterization

The nondominant hand immobilizes the penis with the foreskin pulled back and lifts the shaft.

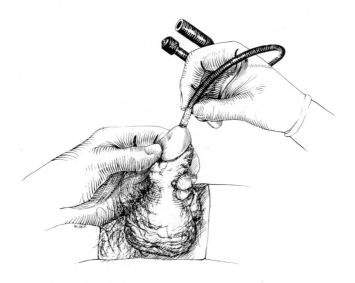

The catheter is passed deep into the bladder to make sure the balloon is not in the urethra. The balloon is inflated to 5 cc (usually) and secured by pulling back until the balloon engages the neck of the bladder.

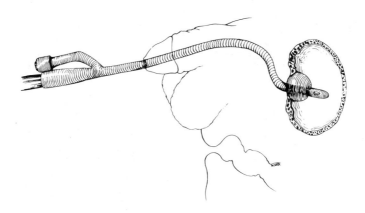

The catheter is connected to a sterile closed collecting system and taped to the thigh. Do not pin or secure the drainage tubing to the bedding.

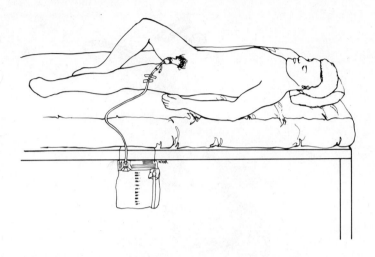

The catheter may be held by a forceps if a nongloved technique is preferred.

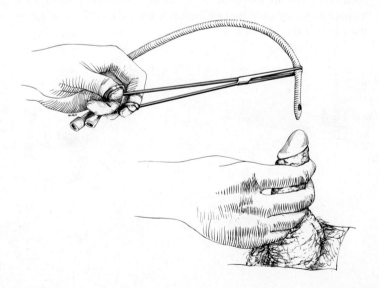

Female Catheterization

The labia are spread to reveal the urethral orifice, which is cleaned with a solution of an aqueous germicide. Prepare *toward* the anus. The catheter is looped in the preferred hand. The thumb and index finger hold the catheter about 2 inches from the tip, and the end is caught between the fourth and fifth fingers.

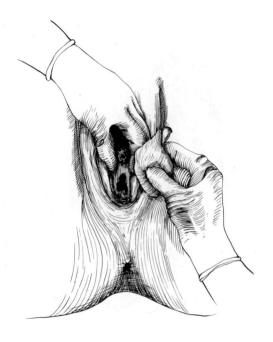

The tip is lubricated and inserted into the orifice. Almost all the catheter is inserted, so that there is no danger of inflating the balloon in the urethra. After the bladder is entered, as indicated by urine flowing from the catheter, the balloon is inflated (usually the 5-cc balloon Foley is used). The catheter is pulled back snugly, secured, and connected to a sterile collecting system.

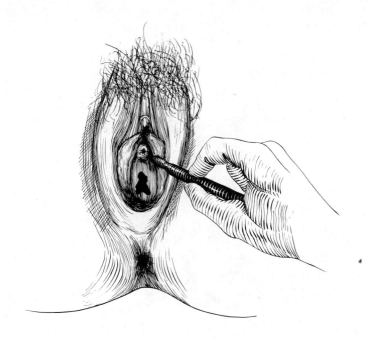

Suprapubic Catheterization

The bladder can be aspirated by a suprapubic technique. Percussion of the abdomen will reveal the level of the bladder. It is hazardous to attempt suprapubic catheterization on a bladder that is not at least moderately distended.

The abdomen is shaved and prepared locally. A 14-gauge intracath should be used. The needle is inserted just above the pubis until the bladder is entered (A). The small catheter is passed through the needle into the bladder (B).

The needle is withdrawn and the catheter is sutured or taped to the skin and connected to a sterile collecting system.

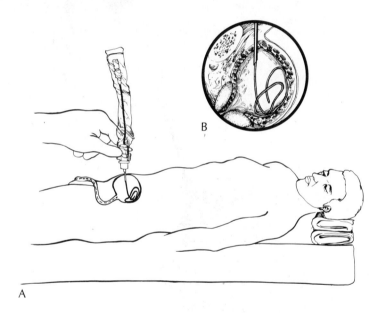

B

A

URETHRAL SOUNDING AND DILATION

For urethral sounding and dilation the penis is held in the same manner as used in catheterization. The glans is cleaned with an aqueous antiseptic. The sound is lubricated with a water-soluble lubricant. A sound smaller than 18F should be used with extreme caution; if a smaller size is required, filiform and follower catheters are safer. A topical anesthetic is often helpful. It should be instilled several minutes before the procedure and retained with a penile clamp.

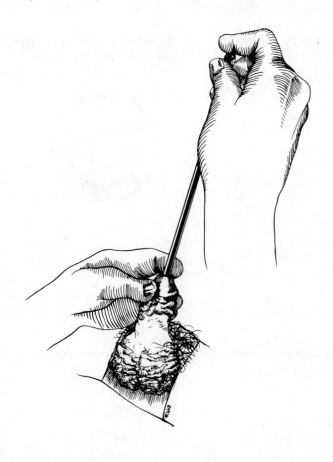

The tip of the sound is advanced as the penis is stabilized. The sound is held parallel to the abdomen.

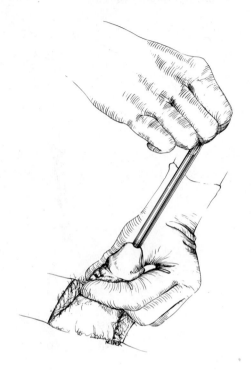

The sound is passed toward the prostate. Then the handle is depressed as the instrument is advanced smoothly. No force should be used lest the urethra be torn.

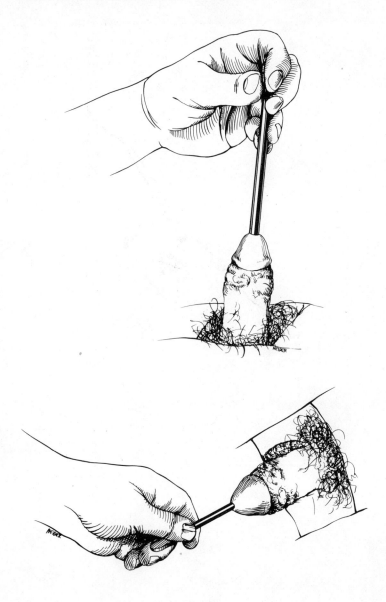

With severe strictures, it may be necessary to insert filiforms and following catheters or sounds. If an obstruction is encountered, the first filiform catheter is left in place and then successive catheters are passed alongside the first until the bladder is entered. The superfluous filiform catheters are then removed.

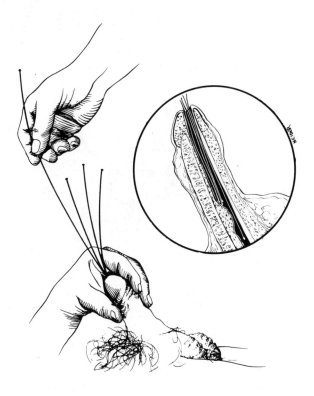

A following sound (LaForte) is connected to the filiform.

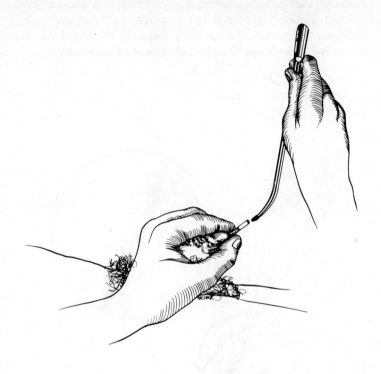

The filiform and follower together are inserted into the bladder. A finger in the rectum may be necessary to guide the sound into the bladder.

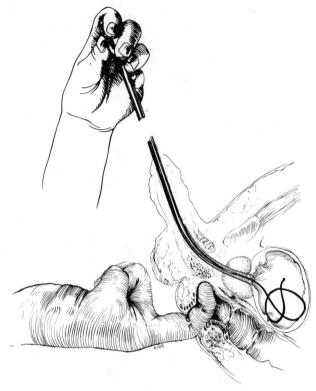

If the sound cannot pass the stricture, detach the follower and leave the filiform in place taped to the penis. Some urine will escape alongside the filiform, decompressing the bladder. After several days the stricture may have softened enough to allow the filiform and follower to enter the bladder.

Never pass more than two or three successive sounds at one time. Further dilation may be necessary and should be repeated at intervals of several weeks or months or more, depending on how rapidly the stricture re-forms.

After each session of sounding, the patient should be on a urinary tract antibiotic for several days. If the sounding was at all difficult, the patient should be held for observation to check on extravasation of urine or bleeding.

A following catheter may be used if bladder drainage is indicated. The screw tip on the catheter is connected to the filiform.

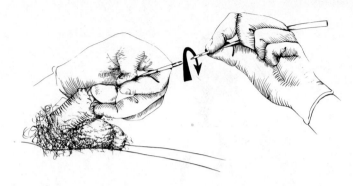

The catheter guided by the filiform is advanced into the bladder to drain the urine.

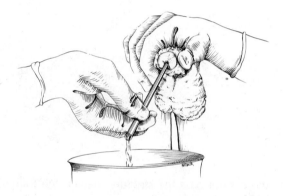

The catheter is secured in position by taping it to the penis.

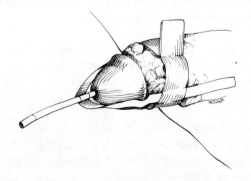

DORSAL SLIT

After shaving, preparing, and draping, the foreskin is anesthetized at the incision site and crushed in a straight clamp 1 cm distal to the corona (A). The tissue is incised with a straight scissors, making sure not to enter the meatus (B, C). Active bleeders are ligated with fine catgut, and the wound margins are approximated using a running suture of 3-0 catgut, taking small bites (D).

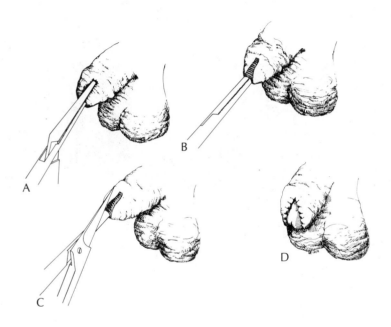

REDUCTION OF PARAPHIMOSIS

Acute swelling of the retracted foreskin should be reduced as soon as possible. Paraphimosis is extremely painful and sedation may be required. Traction on the penile shaft with compression of the glans is performed gently. After reducing the paraphimosis a dorsal slit may be necessary.

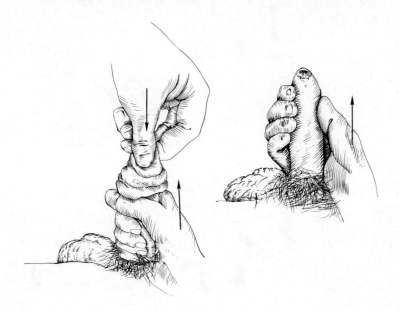

If simple manual reduction is not possible, an incision may be necessary. In this instance, the incision is made dorsally without crushing the skin. Sutures will secure hemostasis. Local anesthesia should be employed.

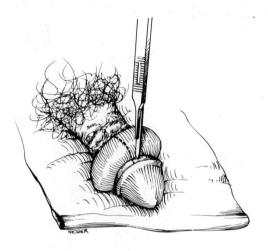

MEATOTOMY

Under local anesthesia, meatal stricture is corrected by inserting a straight arterial clamp and crushing the part of the glans to be opened.

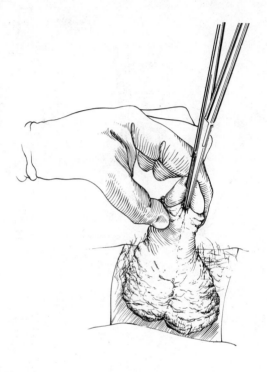

The crushed tissue is opened with a scissors.

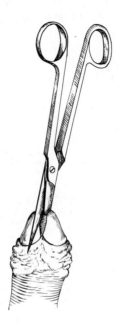

Sutures of 3-0 chromic catgut are used to control bleeding and coapt the tissues.

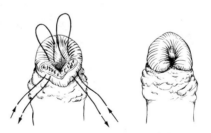

PENILE ANESTHESIA

Anesthesia of the penis can be obtained by infiltrating around the base of the penis using a local anesthetic such as 1% lidocaine. Epinephrine is never used.

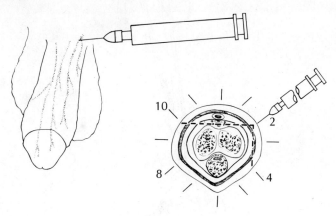

CIRCUMCISION

The suprapubic area and penis are shaved and prepared. Crushing with a straight hemostat provides an avascular area for incision dorsally (A, B). A straight scissors is used to cut the crushed foreskin (C).

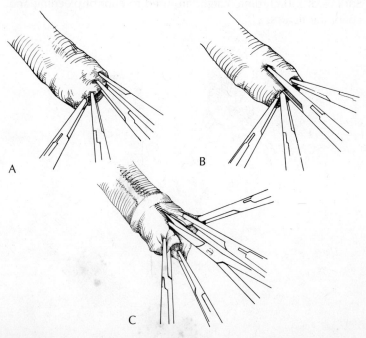

A suture of 3-0 chromic catgut is used to approximate the "mucosa" to the skin at apex of incision (D). The foreskin is cut off with a scissors (E). Individual bleeders are ligated with fine catgut. The tissues are reapproximated with interrupted sutures of 3-0 chromic catgut (F, G). A piece of Vaseline gauze is wrapped around the penis. Then a gauze pad is positioned around the glans and retained with a scrotal support or elastic dressing.

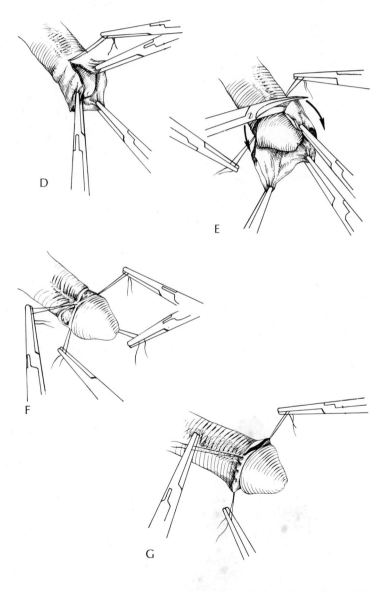

D

E

F

G

URINARY TRACT INJURIES

Examination of the patient with suspected urinary tract injuries should include careful inspection of the abdomen, external genitalia, perineum, rectal area, and bony structures of the pelvis. A careful, gentle rectal examination is performed to evaluate the position and characteristics of the prostate. The condition of the surrounding periprostatic and rectal tissues should be carefully assessed.

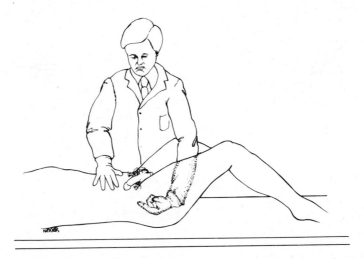

Extravasation of urine due to rupture of any part of the lower urinary tract (bladder, urethra) should be suspected in cases of lower abdominal and pelvic trauma. Generally, injuries involving extravasation of urine are of two distinct types because of the attachment of the urogenital diaphragm to the lateral pelvic walls.

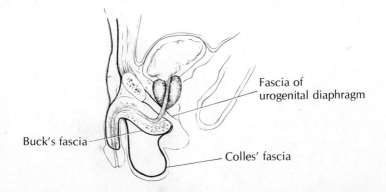

Fascia of
urogenital diaphragm

Buck's fascia

Colles' fascia

If the urethra is torn above the urogenital diaphragm, there may be minimal or no swelling of the penis, scrotum, or upper inner thighs.

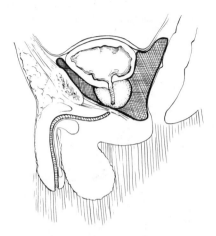

However on rectal examination, the prostate will not be found in the usual position, but may be elevated almost out of reach. A fluctuant or boggy sensation will be present in the periprostatic anterior rectal space.

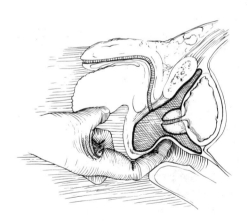

A urethra lacerated below the pelvic diaphragm produces marked swelling or ecchymosis of the penis, scrotum, and perineal areas. This condition should be suspected in the typical "straddle" type of injury. Inspect the perineum carefully for ecchymosis even though swelling may not be present.

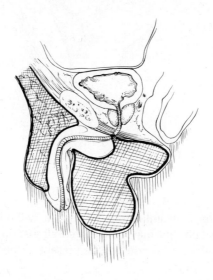

Urethrogram-Cystogram

If an injury to the urethra is suspected, a urethrogram should be performed prior to catheterization. The tip of a genitourinary syringe is held firmly in the urethral meatus, and contrast medium is injected gently. Neomycin should be added.

Integrity of the bladder is confirmed (after the urethrogram) by catheterization of the urethra with a No. 14 or No. 16 Foley catheter. The rubber bulb is removed from the syringe and 250 to 300 ml of contrast medium is poured into the syringe. The catheter is clamped, and anteroposterior and oblique roentgenograms are made. The bladder is then emptied, and the anteroposterior view is repeated to ensure that extravasated contrast medium was not concealed by the bladder shadow.

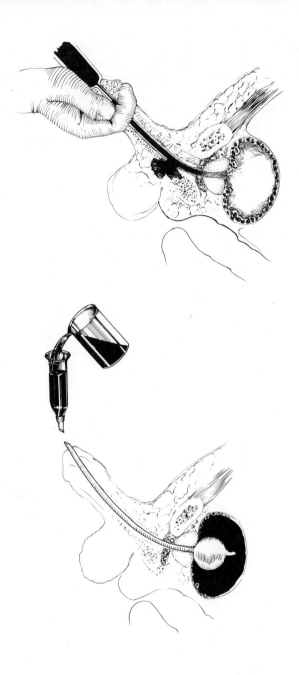

It should also be emphasized that although examination and some diagnostic procedures are performed on an outpatient basis as an emergency basis—or in the emergency department preparatory to admission of the patient—even the most minor injuries to the urethra, whether they are of the infradiaphragmatic or supradiaphragmatic variety, must be managed on an inpatient basis. These injuries are prone to severe complications even under the best of circumstances.

Penile Lacerations
After the usual preparation of the area, minor wounds of the penis, skin or fascial layers are debrided and closed in layers with 3-0 chromic catgut. Antibiotics may be employed for several days subsequently.

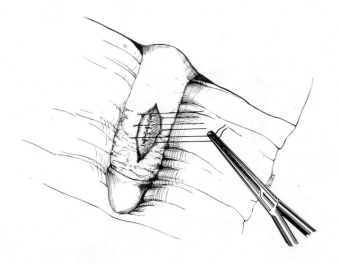

Scrotal Lacerations

Minor wounds of the scrotum are debrided and the layers may be closed with a double layer of interrupted catgut (A, B). A dry dressing is held by a scrotal support. An ice bag may give some relief, and the patient should remain at home in bed for 24 to 48 hours. Antibiotics should be employed for several days afterward. A small Penrose drain may be left in place for a day or two if much oozing occurs.

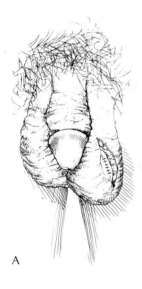

A

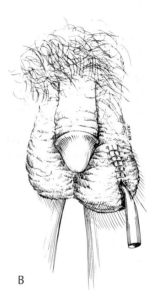

B

VASECTOMY

The penis and scrotum are shaved and prepared. The ductus deferens is identified by palpation and held between the thumb and forefinger (A). The area is infiltrated with a local anesthetic, and a small incision is made over the area.

The ductus is isolated by blunt dissection from the other cord sutures (B). Two nonabsorbable sutures are placed approximately 1 inch apart (C). A 1- to 2-cm section is removed (D).

The ends of the ductus may be doubled back and tied again with 2-0 silk suture (E). All the layers of the scrotum are closed with one or two 3-0 catgut sutures (F).

A dry gauze dressing is held with a scrotal support. Wait for 5 to 10 minutes and observe for delayed bleeding. A scrotal support is recommended for a few days. The patient must be reminded that sterility will not be achieved for at least 4 to 6 weeks. A sample of ejaculate at that time must be examined microscopically to confirm azoospermia.

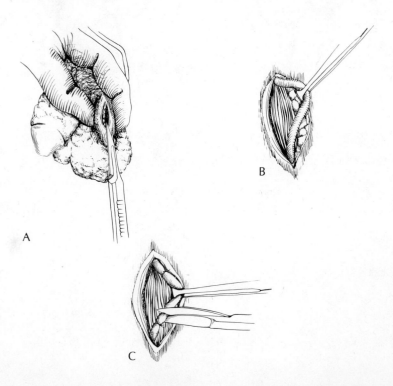

A

B

C

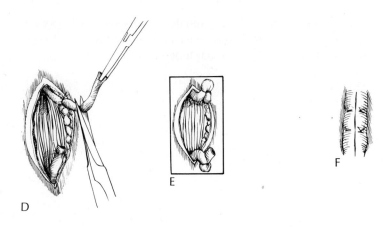

D

E

F

PERINEAL NEEDLE BIOPSY OF THE PROSTATE

The patient is placed in the lithotomy position on the cystoscopy table with the legs elevated. The table may be placed in slight Trendelenburg position.

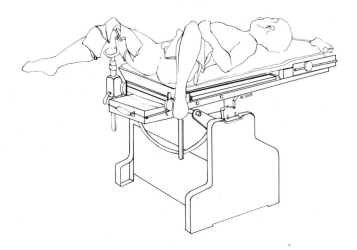

The perineum is shaved and prepared, and a local anesthetic is injected by first raising a skin wheal and infiltrating the tissues in the midline between the ischial tuberosities.

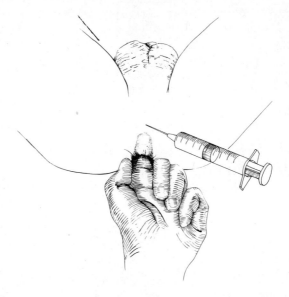

The site of the skin wheal is incised with a No. 11 blade, and a needle of the Vim-Silverman type is introduced and guided into the prostatic nodule by the rectal finger.

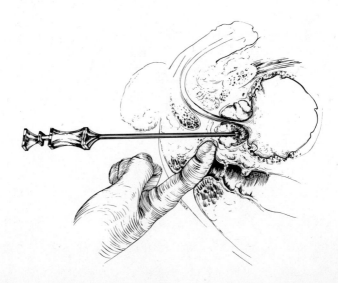

REMOVAL OF STRANGULATING OBJECTS FROM THE PENIS

Heavy twine is wrapped circumferentially around the penile shaft 3 to 4 cm distal to the object (A). A small hemostat is passed underneath the object, grasping the loose proximal end of the cord (B). This end is slowly unwound, milking out the edema fluid as the ring is removed (C). The procedure may need to be repeated, and lubricating the area with mineral oil may be helpful.

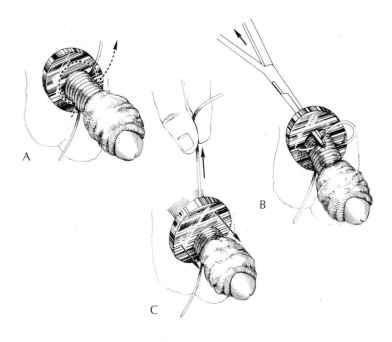

A

B

C

12

Obstetrics and Gynecology

H. Marvin Camel

The diseases and functional problems of the human female contribute heavily to the ever-increasing patient population in the emergency and outpatient areas of most hospitals. Many of these patients present with lower abdominal complaints, many of which are the result of lower genital tract infections. It must never be forgotten, however, that mild pain can presage the onset of many life-threatening conditions, and a complete, appropriate history and physical examination are therefore required for each patient. Always question the patient carefully about her menstrual cycle, keeping in mind the possibility of pregnancy in any woman of childbearing age. To avoid the possibility of producing a fetal malformation, pregnancy must be excluded before roentgenograms of the abdomen are made or certain drugs ordered.

Examinations
ABDOMEN
The general examination of the abdomen is considered elsewhere, but certain points specifically relevant to the female abdomen must be emphasized.

A slight prominence of the area between the umbilicus and symphysis, noted in inspecting the abdomen, may be the result of a distended bladder, enlarging uterus, or beginning paralytic ileus from bacterial peritonitis or blood in the pelvis. Scars of prior surgical procedures must be noted, and it must not be assumed that just because a hysterectomy has been done, the appendix was removed at that same time. It should also be noted whether or not the pubic hair distribution is that of a normal female. Abnormal patterns may give a clue to adrenal or ovarian tumors.

The usual palpations, percussions, and auscultations are done as in any other patient, whether adult or child. Always ask the patient to use one finger to indicate the point of maximal pain. If the patient's finger moves immediately to one point and stays, this is more significant than if it moves in and out all across the lower abdomen.

URINE CULTURE
Before the pelvic organs are examined, the patient should empty her bladder, and a midstream specimen should be collected by the clean catch technique as follows: The patient holds the labia apart, and the urethral orifice is wiped with an antiseptic sponge. Only after the bladder has been partially emptied is the specimen bottle filled with urine.

A patient with urinary retention should be checked for a retained vaginal tampon. If the vagina is clear, pregnancy, or a psycho-neurotic problem, or both must be considered. Suprapubic aspiration by a sterile intravenous plastic catheter (Chap. 11) is safer than passing a urethral catheter to empty the bladder only once.

PELVIC EXAMINATION
Before the speculum, or gloved fingers, or both are introduced, time must be taken to inspect the external genitalia, including the pubic area and inner thighs. Bruises, scratches, swelling, and any discharges should all be sought and noted carefully. A purulent discharge should be followed back to its origin by spreading the labia gently and observing the various orifices. A smear and culture of any purulent material must be made as the initial step in patient care. The urethral orifice and cervical os must be cultured, checking for gonorrhea; with another swab, the anal canal should be sampled, avoiding too deep penetration, which could cause fecal contamination. Gonorrhea must be excluded in any female who presents with the complaints of dysuria and or lower abdominal pains.

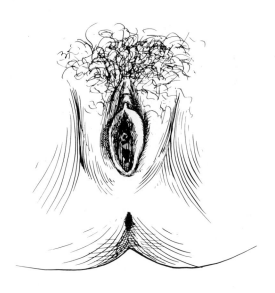

Speculum Examination

The internal female genitalia are examined by the use of the speculum, followed by manual examination. The tray is pictured as it is usually prepared for this procedure.

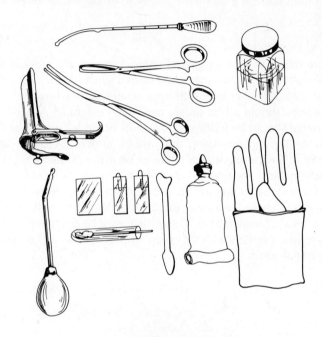

It is best to lubricate the speculum only with warm water. Many lubricants contain antiseptics or antibiotics that will interfere with obtaining a culture of the bacterial flora of the cervix and vagina. The labia are spread gently with the left hand, the urethral orifice is exposed, and a sample taken. Then the speculum is introduced and the blades opened slowly and gently. A swab sample is taken from the cervical os and from the posterior vaginal pool. The swab should be plated immediately or introduced into a suitable transport culture medium. Another swab of the posterior vaginal pool may be streaked on a slide for a Gram stain. An aspirate of the vaginal pool can be placed on a slide, covered with a coverslip, and examined for mobile trichomonads if a *Trichomonas* infection is suspected; or the swab is placed in 1 ml of saline and the resultant suspension examined for mobile forms.

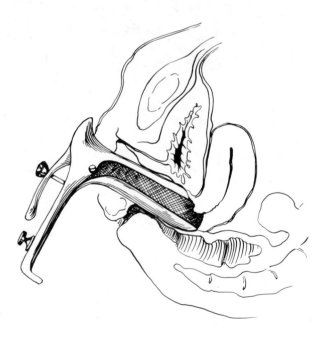

Bimanual Examination

One examining finger is introduced initially along the posterior vaginal wall to the cervix, which is moved posteriorly, then side to side. While performing the pelvic examination, it is well to keep talking to the patient to distract her and help her to relax. Pain elicited on any motion of the cervix is very suggestive of pelvic peritonitis.

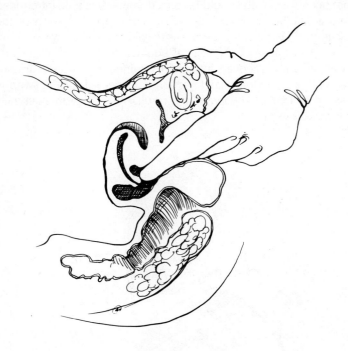

After the initial one-finger examination, bimanual examination of the adnexal areas is next performed. Rectovaginal or rectal examination (or both) is performed only after changing the glove of that hand to prevent the possible introduction of gonorrhea into the anal canal. An accurate determination of the size of the uterus can only be done on rectal examination.

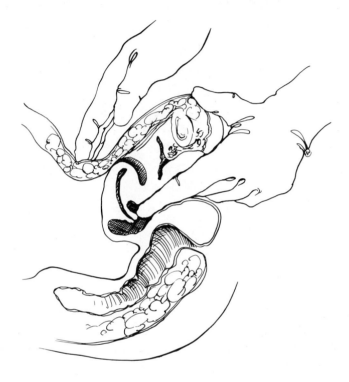

Laboratory Studies

PAPANICOLAOU EXAMINATION. In the Papanicolaou examination, the broad blade pictured scrapes the vaginal pool and is smeared on one slide. The opposite tip is designed to be inserted into the cervical os. The spatula is twisted 360°, and the material is smeared on another slide. Both slides are immediately immersed in a container filled with 50 to 95% alcohol and 50% ether.

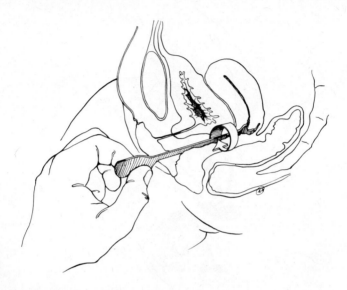

TEST FOR YEASTS AND FUNGI. To test for the presence of yeasts and fungi, vaginal material is spread on a slide, and two drops of 10% KOH solution are added to the wet slide. The slide is examined in 5 minutes for mycelia and spores.

GRAM STAIN. For Gram stains, the vaginal material is smeared on the slide, and the slide is heated gently to fix. The slide is then covered with Gram's crystal violet stain for 1 minute, and a few drops of bicarbonate solution are added. The slide is then washed, covered with Gram's iodine solution for 1 minute, decolorized with ether acetone solution for 1 second, and washed immediately. It is then flooded with safranine dye for 1 minute, dried, and examined.

SCHILLER TEST. Normal cervical squamous cells contain glycogen and stain brown when the area is painted with Gram's iodine solution. One should suspect the presence of atypical cells in areas of no staining. These are the sites where a biopsy should be done.

BIOPSY OF CERVIX. If there are multiple areas which do not stain by the Schiller technique or if multiple erosions are present, the patient usually needs to be admitted to the hospital for conization of the cervix and study of the entire specimen.

Small biopsy specimens may be obtained with a cup biopsy forceps. Specimens may be taken from several areas in one procedure.

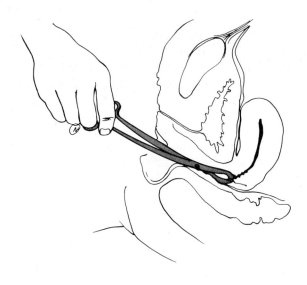

ENDOMETRIAL BIOPSY. Endometrial biopsy is frequently done to evaluate the endometrial status and to time ovulation. The small biopsy instrument that is used is inserted through the cervical os to the depth of the fundus. Then, as it is withdrawn, suction is applied and the tip samples the uterine endometrium. The specimen obtained is placed in 10% formalin solution for pathologic examination.

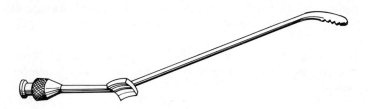

CERVICAL MUCUS ARBORIZATION ("FERNING"). When cervical mucus is spread and allowed to dry for 10 minutes on a glass slide, a fernlike pattern forms when the sample is obtained during the seventh to the eighteenth day of a normal menstrual cycle.

AMNIOTIC FLUID FERNING. Amniotic fluid from a ruptured amniotic sac, when allowed to dry on a slide, also produces a fern pattern. Amniotic fluid also turns nitrazine paper blue, indicating an alkaline pH.

Uterine Malposition

RETROFLEXION AND RETROVERSION

In first-degree retroflexion, the uterus is flexed posteriorly on the cervix, so that the cervix is tipped only slightly posteriorly (A). In second-degree retroflexion, the body of the uterus and cervix are almost in a straight line (B). In retroversion, the cervix and the entire body are tipped posteriorly, so that the cervix presents in an anterior position in the vagina (C). Retroflexion or retroversion are seldom the source of pelvic symptoms, although the associated position of the ovaries in the cul de sac may contribute to dyspareunia.

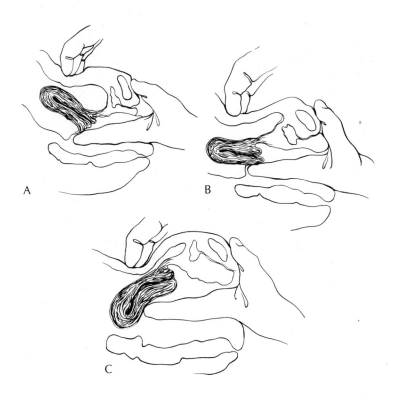

A

B

C

MANUAL REDUCTION OF UTERINE MALPOSITION

An attempt can be made to return the body of the uterus to its normal relation with the cervix. If the retroplacement can be corrected manually, a pessary may be inserted by a physician trained in this procedure. Relaxations of the pelvic floor and the various degrees of uterine prolapse and their management are beyond the scope of this discussion.

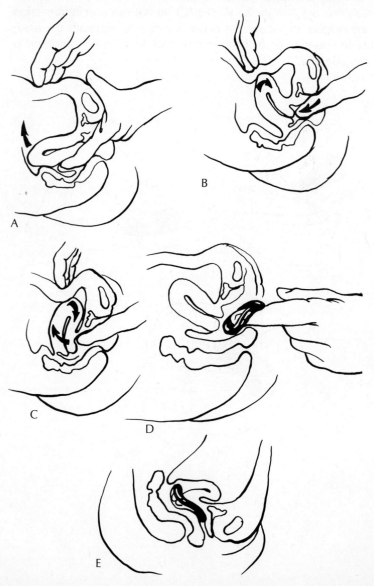

A

B

C

D

E

Pregnancy and Associated Conditions
SIGNS OF PREGNANCY

Personnel who work primarily in the emergency and outpatient areas of hospitals are frequently called on to diagnose and manage some aspects of pregnancy. The determination that the patient is pregnant can be made with considerable reliability by submitting a urine sample to the laboratory. However, there are a number of clinical signs that customarily are used to confirm pregnancy.

Presumptive Signs
1. Absence of menstruation in excess of 15 days past the expected date of onset.
2. Nausea and vomiting.
3. Enlargement and "tingling" of the breasts, with development of Montgomery's follicles around the areola.
4. Increased vaginal discharge of white cells and mucus.
5. Increased frequency of urination and decreased amounts of urine, resulting from pressure on the bladder by the enlarging uterus.

Probable Signs
1. The pregnant uterus softens, especially at the junction point between the cervix and fundus (Hegar's sign).
2. The cervix and vagina become more bluish as a result of the increasing vascularity of the pelvic organs (Chadwick's sign).
3. Enlargement of the uterus out of the pelvis normally occurs after the second month.

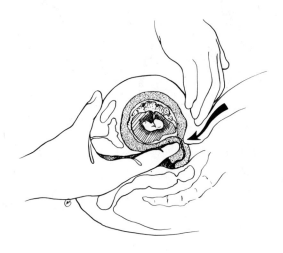

Positive Signs

The positive signs of pregnancy include fetal movement, a placental souffle on auscultation, a fetal skeleton on x-ray examination, and a fetal heartbeat.

ESTIMATING THE DURATION OF PREGNANCY

The usual pregnancy requires 10 lunar months of 28 days, or 280 days, but there is considerable variation on both sides of this figure. The duration of a pregnancy can be estimated by measuring the size of the uterus, assuming a normal pregnancy in a normal woman:

Fourth month: Four fingers above the symphysis.
Fifth month: Halfway between the symphysis and umbilicus.
Sixth month: At the umbilicus.
Seventh month: Three fingers above the umbilicus.
Ninth month: Almost at the xiphoid process.

After the sixth month, the lunar month of the pregnancy can be determined by measuring the distance from the top of the fundus to the cephalad surface of the symphysis with a tape measure. The distance measured in centimeters is divided by 3.5 to find the month. This is called McDonald's rule.

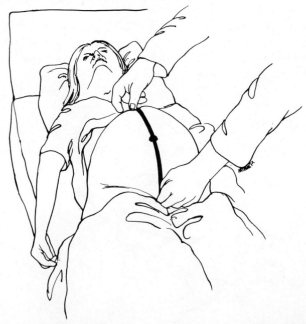

PROLAPSED CORD

If the patient arrives in the emergency department with a pro-lapsed umbilical cord, it should be checked for pulsations. Absence of pulsations and of fetal heart tones indicates that the fetus is dead and no emergency exists. If, on the other hand, the cord is still pulsating, two fingers must be inserted into the vagina, with the cord between, to keep the descending head from compress-ing the cord. The patient must be taken at once to the delivery suite with a physician or nurse protecting the cord in this fashion.

DELIVERY

Pelvic measurements and the management of the prenatal pa-tient are not within the purview of this book, nor are the compli-cations of pregnancy or unusual presentations. However, the pregnant patient may arrive at the hospital in such an advanced stage of labor as to preclude her being taken to the delivery suite.

Labor

Labor is customarily divided into three stages:

FIRST STAGE. The first stage begins with the onset of painful con-tractions, usually accompanied by the passage of blood-tinged mucus ("bloody show"), and lasts until the cervix is thinned out (effacement) and dilated. At this point, the membranes custom-arily rupture, i.e., the "bag of water" breaks.

SECOND STAGE. In the second stage of labor the infant descends through the pelvis. The patient bears down involuntarily, and the stretched perineum bulges. This stage ends when the infant is born.

THIRD STAGE. After the infant is born, the contractions cease for a few minutes, then recommence until the placenta is delivered, terminating the third and final stage.

Emergency Department Management

DELIVERY OF THE INFANT. Customarily, the infant is facing the mother's right side (the examiner's left), and, as the head passes through the pelvis, the head turns on the shoulders to allow the occiput to pass under the symphysis.

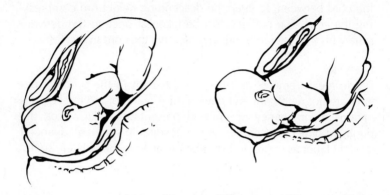

It may be helpful for the person delivering the infant to aid in extension of the head by upward pressure, with the draped hand pushing back the mother's rectum. As soon as the head is delivered, if the cord is around the neck, it must be slipped over the head to avoid (1) strangling the baby, or (2) avulsing the placenta, or (3) producing inversion of the uterus. If the cord cannot be slipped over the head, it must be doubly clamped and sectioned.

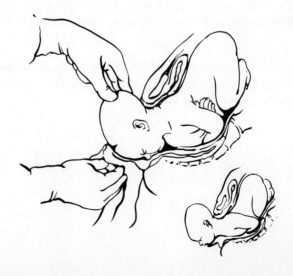

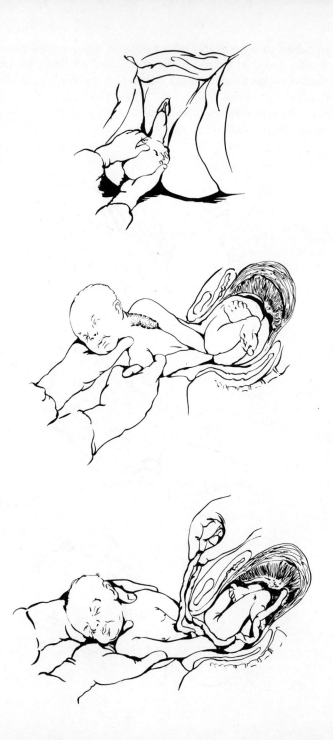

After the baby's head has been delivered, mucus must be aspirated from the mouth and nose, especially from the latter, since babies are nose breathers.

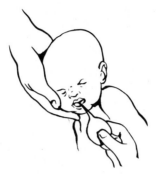

Episiotomy is a delivery suite procedure, but if it is obvious that the perineum is about to tear, a posterior lateral or midline incision is made with a scissors.

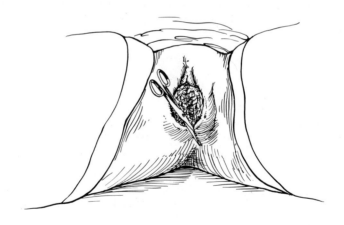

After delivery, the baby is placed on the mother's abdomen, and when the pulsations have ceased, the cord is doubly clamped and sectioned. If the child is erythroblastotic or needs cardiopulmonary resuscitation, the cord is cut between clamps immediately after the delivery. The child is wrapped in a blanket, and a drop of 1% silver nitrate is placed in each eye to prevent ophthalmia neonatorum. The eyes are then irrigated with saline.

DELIVERY OF THE PLACENTA. Expulsion of the placenta is aided by massaging the fundus of the uterus or even squeezing the fundus through the flaccid abdominal wall (Credé's maneuver). The placenta must be inspected after delivery to ensure complete expulsion.

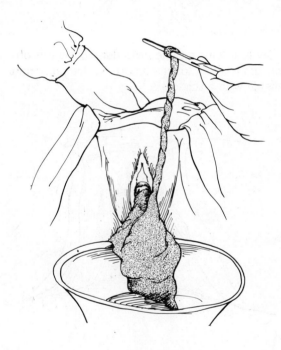

If an episiotomy was made, it is usually closed in the delivery suite with a running 3-0 catgut suture. The skin is closed in a subcuticular manner, and the end is caught in a shot.

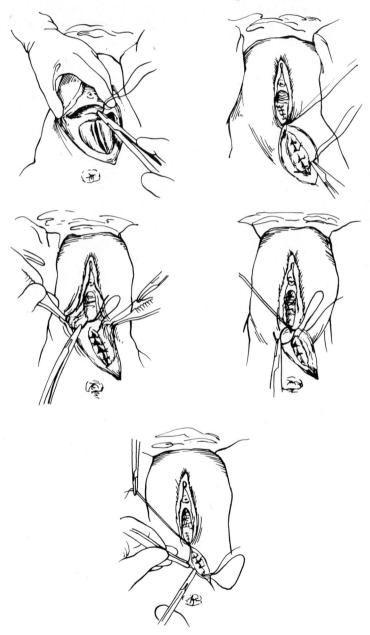

PUDENDAL BLOCK. Anesthesia for the episiotomy repair or even for the delivery, if time permits, is obtained by pudendal block; 10 to 20 ml of 1% lidocaine is infiltrated around the nerve as it passes adjacent to the ischial spine on each side. The syringe and needle are guided by one finger in the vagina, and the needle is inserted toward the spines through the vaginal wall.

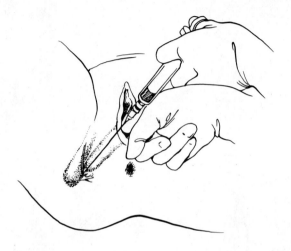

APGAR SCORE. An infant delivered in the emergency department is usually in excellent condition, for there has been no time to administer any narcotics or anesthetics to the mother, which would depress the infant's activity. The Apgar Test, devised by the anesthesiologist Virginia Apgar, is used to evaluate the infant's physical status. The maximal score is 10, determined as shown in Table 12-1, which also provides a device to aid the memory.

Table 12-1. Apgar Scoring

Sign	Score		
	0	1	2
Color (A = anoxia)	Blue, pale	Body, pink; extremities, blue	Completely pink
Heart (P = pulse)	Absent	Below 100	Over 100
Reflex irritability (catheter in nostril) (G = grimace)	None	Grimace	Good, crying
Muscle tone (A = activity)	Limp	Some flexion of extremities	Active motion
Respiratory effort (R = respiratory)	Absent	Irregular	Cough, sneeze

ABORTION

Spontaneous Abortion

The patient who has missed a menstrual period by more than 15 days and then begins to pass blood can be managed by bed rest, possibly in a hospital on an obstetric service. It is doubtful that this will prevent abortion, but the restricted activity is traditional.

However, on occasion, the patient may be passing clots and bleeding heavily. (*Note:* The patient's statement that she is passing "liver" = clots; "hamburger" = placenta.) When she presents in the emergency department, she should be positioned on the table and a vaginal speculum inserted gently.

If the cervix is dilated and tissue is extruding, a ring forceps is used to remove it.

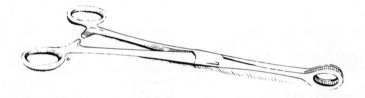

Induced Abortion: Suction Curettage

Evacuation of the pregnant uterus in the first 3 months is accomplished by the suction catheter technique.

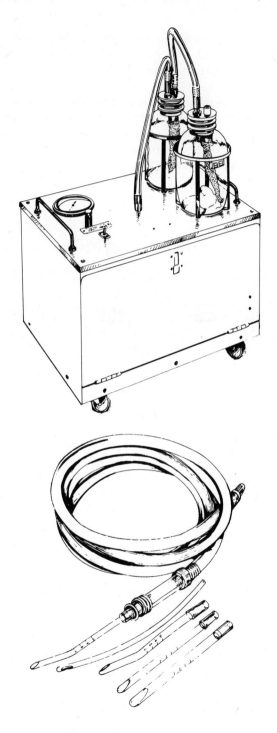

Obstetrics and Gynecology **335**

The vagina is prepared in the usual fashion, and a sterile speculum is inserted. The suction tip is gently inserted to the fundus, and the suction motor is started.

As the catheter is withdrawn, it removes the fetus. The motor is then stopped while the catheter is reinserted, and the procedure is repeated until no further tissue is obtained. The collection bottle must be checked to make sure that the fetus and membranes are completely removed.

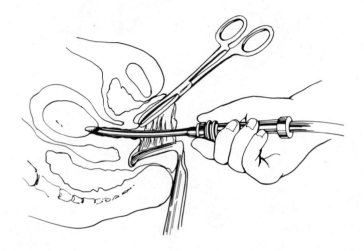

The patient should be kept in bed for 2 to 4 hours to make sure no hemorrhage occurs. If it does not, she is discharged, but her activities should be limited for a few days thereafter.

CULDOCENTESIS

If a patient is suspected of having an intraabdominal hemorrhage (frequently from a ruptured ectopic pregnancy), aspiration of the abdominal cavity may be done through the posterior vaginal fornix. The procedure may also be done to aspirate purulent material for culture and sensitivity testing in cases of pelvis peritonitis.

The vagina is held open with a sterile speculum and swabbed with an antiseptic. The posterior lip of the cervix is grasped with a tenaculum and steadied. A No. 18 spinal needle connected to a syringe is inserted through the posterior vaginal fornix. Suction is applied by the syringe while this is done.

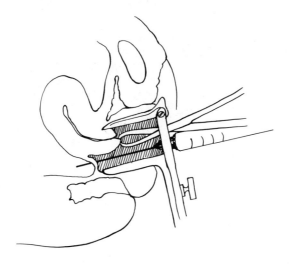

If the blood that is obtained does not clot in 4 to 6 minutes or contains shreds of clots, the diagnosis of an intraabdominal hemorrhage is confirmed. If serosanguinous material is obtained, the possibility exists that an ovarian cyst has ruptured, causing the symptoms. In this instance, careful observation may be all the patient needs.

The aspiration of purulent material in a septic patient is an ominous sign that a tubo-ovarian abscess has ruptured. Purulent material should be cultured, smeared, and stained and the patient prepared for laparotomy.

Problems of the Introitus

IMPERFORATE HYMEN

The girl with an imperforated hymen is usually brought to the physician because of amenorrhea. If amenorrhea has been present long enough, an abdominal mass may be palpable. The mass is the distended uterus filled with retained menstrual products. Characteristically, the bulging hymen presents itself at the introitus. A simple linear incision can be made without anesthesia.

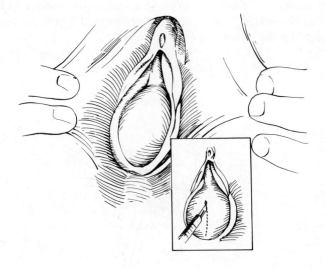

HYMENEAL HEMORRHAGE

Infrequently, the first penetration of the vagina results in significant bleeding from the ruptured hymen, and it is not uncommon for the embarrassed couple to wait until a considerable amount of blood has been lost before coming to the hospital. The bleeding point is usually easily identified, and a 3-0 catgut suture with or without local anesthesia will control the problem.

Ordinarily, as soon as the head has been delivered it rotates to one side, and then the rest of the body rapidly follows. This can be aided by gentle downward traction on the head to impinge the anterior shoulder beneath the pubis. The head is then lifted toward the symphysis, so that the posterior shoulder is delivered. Completion of the delivery quickly follows.

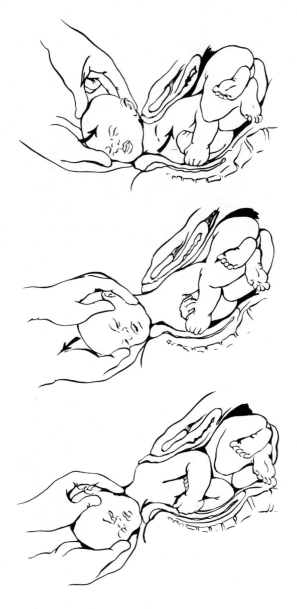

BARTHOLIN CYSTS OR ABSCESSES

Bartholin cysts result from obstruction of a Bartholin's gland duct, with infection frequently superimposed. The uninfected cyst may be removed in toto in the hospital, but the infected cyst is best drained and cultured, with definitive treatment delayed. Such cysts usually occur in the labia minora but also may involve the labia majora (A).

The cyst is drained as follows: A small amount of 1% lidocaine injected in the projected incision site provides local anesthesia (B). The incision should be made on the medial side toward the introitus and should be large enough to be kept open easily. The walls of the cyst are sutured with 3-0 catgut to the walls of the opening in the labia (C). By this means, excision may be avoided, for the large permanent opening can drain easily.

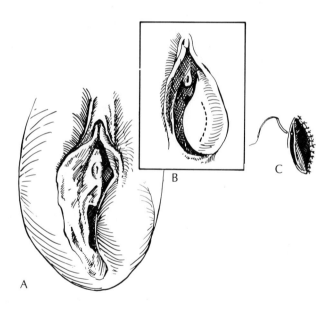

CONDYLOMA ACUMINATUM

Condylomata acuminata of the perineum are common and result from a virus that accompanies leukorrhea and must be corrected simultaneously.

A mixture of 25% podophyllum (7.5 gm of podophyllum in 1 ounce of tincture benzoin compound) can be applied to the warty growths after a thick coat of Vaseline has been applied over the normal areas to prevent burning of this skin. The area may be washed after 2 to 3 hours. This treatment can be repeated at weekly intervals until the lesions completely disappear.

Condylomata may be removed under local or under general anesthesia by electrofulguration at one or more sessions, depending on the extent of the lesions. Destruction by a cryoprobe is also effective.

Rape

The personnel who handle the victim of rape must do so with great gentleness and kindness, remembering that the woman has had a very traumatic experience. Squads of policewomen have been established in many cities to aid in rape investigations. These women are trained to handle the rape victim sympathetically and not to adopt the attitude of many officials that the victim is making unjustified accusations or that the attack was provoked by her behavior or what she was wearing.

MANAGEMENT

The patient's remarks about the attacks must be carefully recorded. The examiner must avoid the diagnosis of "alleged rape," which is construed by juries to mean that the examining physician does not believe that rape occurred. The mental attitudes and general behavior of the patient should be described. The woman's clothing must be examined to see if it is torn, and her entire body must be examined for bruises and scratches. The perineal area, inner thighs, and introitus must be carefully inspected for abrasions, ecchymoses, and lacerations. A fine-tooth comb must be passed through the pubic and labial hairy areas and the retained hairs sealed in a carefully marked envelope, to be turned over to the police.

A speculum is lubricated only with a small amount of water and then passed gently into the vagina, again in a search for tears and abrasions. The vaginal vault is aspirated with a small bulb syringe, and the following steps are then taken:

1. The material is placed on a slide as a hanging drip and examined for spermatozoa.
2. If active sperm are found, a small amount is sent to the laboratory to determine the blood type of the sperm.
3. If no sperm are seen and yet the material appears to be seminal fluid, the material may be sent to the laboratory to test for acid phosphatase.
4. A smear of the cervix and vagina should be taken, placed in broth, sent to the bacteriology laboratory for culture and sensitivity, and smeared on special media for gonorrhea. The patient may be offered prophylactic treatment for gonorrhea. The antibiotic dosages are the same as those used in culture proved cases. At the present time penicillin is most commonly used.

1. Penicillin G, 4.8 million units (2.4 million units in each hip), with 1 gm of oral probenecid.
2. Ampicillin, 3.5 gm orally, with 1 gm of oral probenecid.
3. Tetracycline, 1.5 gm orally immediately; then 0.5 gm orally four times a day for 4 days.
4. Spectinomycin, 4.0 gm intramuscularly.

If the patient has no religious objections, she should be offered contraception. Diethylstilbestrol is commonly used (i.e., 25 mg given orally twice a day for 5 days). This may induce some nausea, but will probably produce a menstrual flow after the medication is stopped, thereby preventing the implantation of a fertilized ovum. An intrauterine device may be inserted.

If diethylstilbestrol does not produce a menstrual period, the uterus must be mechanically evacuated to avoid the possibility of adenocarcinoma of the vagina later in life should the fetus be a female.

13

Anus and Rectum
Outpatient Procedures

Charles B. Anderson

Many procedures, both diagnostic and therapeutic, can be performed in the emergency department to investigate and alleviate anorectal problems. The ability to complete these procedures expeditiously and carefully will prevent unnecessary hospitalization. It is essential to recognize that certain kinds of treatment demand hospitalization and should await the patient's admission to the hospital.

Biopsies of the sigmoid colon or rectum above the peritoneal reflection pose the risk of free peritoneal perforation if the biopsy is too deep. Prolapse of the rectum requires a complicated surgical approach, and abscesses in the pelvirectal space require incision and drainage under general anesthesia.

Anatomy of the Rectum and Anus

The rectum is approximately 15 cm long and extends proximally from the pectinate line. The anus starts at the pectinate line and is the distal 3.5 cm of the gastrointestinal tract. It joins the rectum at approximately a right angle. The anus is directed anterosuperiorly and the rectum posterosuperior. The mucosa above the pectinate line is supplied by sensory fibers from the autonomic nervous system; the epithelium in the anus has somatic sensory innervation. Therefore, above the pectinate line, there is no sensory response to painful stimuli; below the pectinate line, local anesthesia is required because pain sensation is intact.

The anal glands originate from the anal crypts at the pectinate line. It is from these glands that perirectal infections and fistulas originate. Internal hemorrhoids occur above the pectinate line, external hemorrhoids below it.

The levator ani muscle extends down into the anal area and forms a portion of the anal sphincter. Infections above this muscle lie in the pelvirectal space and require general anesthesia for drainage; infections below it are often deeply placed and also require general anesthesia for drainage. Some infections present in the perianal skin may be drained adequately under local anesthesia on an outpatient basis (see Perirectal Abscess). Longitudinal and circular muscles make up the anal sphincter; it is important not to divide all muscle layers because of possible anal incontinence. However, portions of the sphincter muscles can be divided without complications.

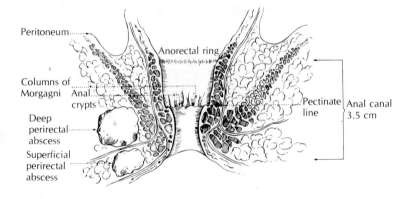

In the male the prostate lies anteriorly and can be adequately examined through the rectum. Above the prostate is the posterior surface of the bladder, and immediately above this area, within reach of the finger, lies the cul-de-sac, where pelvic abscesses occur and point into the anterior rectum.

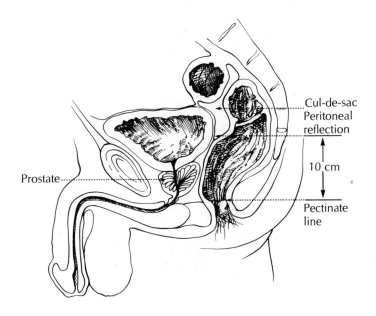

Cul-de-sac
Peritoneal reflection

10 cm

Prostate

Pectinate line

In the female the cervix is palpated through the anterior rectal wall and can be examined in this manner, although somewhat inadequately, when one does not wish to contaminate the vaginal canal, as, for example, during labor, to determine cervical dilatation. Above the cervix of the uterus is the cul-de-sac, as previously described.

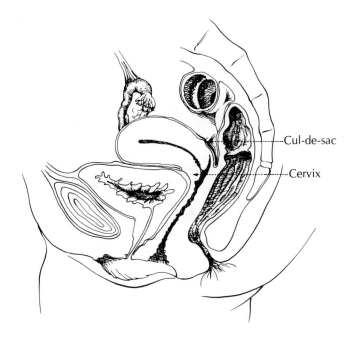

Cul-de-sac

Cervix

Digital Examination

A rectal glove, lubricant jelly, gentleness, careful palpation, and visual inspection are required for a proper examination of the anus and rectum. Although the examination can be made adequately with the patient lying supine in bed with the knees and hips flexed, the patient is best examined in the lithotomy position. The perirectal area is visualized and palpated for abnormal swellings, indicative of abscess, sinus tracts, or fistulas communicating with the rectum.

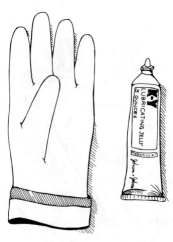

Gentle spreading of the buttocks may identify fissures in the anal area. Bearing down will cause internal hemorrhoids to protrude.

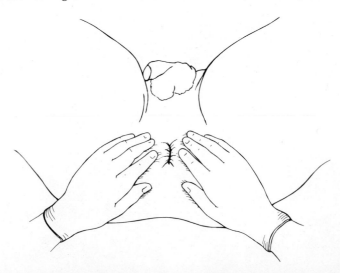

The lubricated finger is inserted into the rectum by applying steady but gentle pressure on the anal orifice. The patient is requested to bear down as if having a bowel movement. Rough and traumatic insertion of the finger will be painful and cause spasm of the anal sphincter. Once the finger is inserted, it is briefly left in position without further movement, to allow the patient to relax. The anterior and lateral walls are palpated for masses, tenderness, and fissures. The cervix of the uterus in females and the prostate in males can be examined at this time. The finger is rotated to both sides and then continued posteriorly to complete circumferential evaluation of the anal canal and lower rectum.

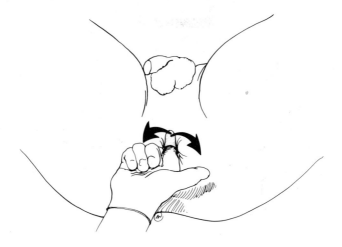

A tender protrusion presenting anteriorly and high in the rectum, often felt only with the patient bearing down strenuously, is usually indicative of an abscess in the cul-de-sac. Aspiration of this area through the rectum may be attempted only after further surgical consultation and admission of the patient to the hospital. Incision and drainage of pelvic abscesses through the rectum is beyond the scope of this discussion.

On withdrawing the finger, a small amount of feces is removed and tested for the presence of occult blood. Special kits are available for this purpose. A thin layer of feces is applied to the center of the card, after which 2 drops of Hemoccult developer (a stabilized solution of hydrogen peroxide and denatured alcohol) are added. A blue color, most easily visible on the white paper, indicates the presence of blood. If blood is discovered, further examination by anoscopy, or sigmoidoscopy, or both and perhaps by barium enema will be required.

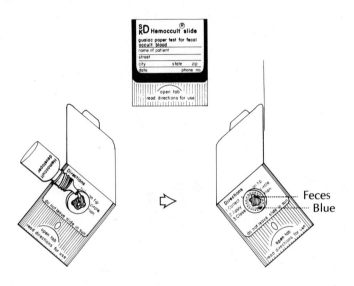

Fractures or dislocations of the coccyx can usually be diagnosed during bidigital examination with the index finger in the rectum and the thumb placed externally posterior to the rectum. Hernias of the obturator canal are also diagnosed by rectal examination.

Anoscopy

Examination of the anus and distal rectum is performed best with an anoscope. One type of instrument consists of an obturator inserted into a cylinder that has a handle to facilitate manipulation.

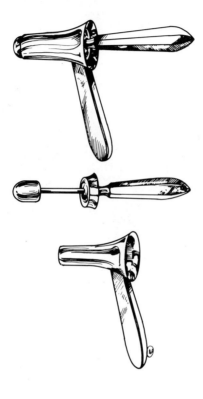

A well-lubricated anoscope is gently inserted into the anus as described for the digital examination. The instrument is inserted anteriorly toward the midline, following the direction of the anal canal (A). The obturator is held in place with the thumb until fully inserted, then the obturator is removed (B). A speculum that permits separation of the blades for wider exposure may also be used (C).

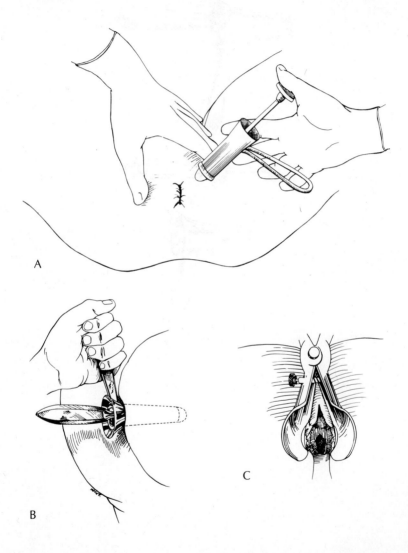

A

B

C

The anoscope is inserted to the maximal extent and then rotated through 360°, so that all quadrants of the anus are inspected. External illumination through a separate light source is required when using this instrument. A fiberoptic light source, a flashlight, or a gooseneck lamp are adequate. Swabs, or suction, or both are needed to keep the area clean. Anal fissures will often cause much pain and may necessitate treatment with a topical anesthetic prior to instrumentation. Anoscopy can usually be performed without enema preparation. The lateral decubitus position will often prove adequate if stirrups are not available for putting the patient in the lithotomy position.

Fistulous tracts, hemorrhoids, polyps, and inflammation (proctitis) are commonly encountered. When foreign bodies are lodged in the rectum, general anesthesia is frequently required for their safe removal.

Sigmoidoscopy

The equipment used in sigmoidoscopy consists of the sigmoidoscope (demonstrated with the obturator in place), an obturator, a round-tipped metal sucker, an electric light source, swabs, and an insufflator that dilates the rectum and facilitates passage of the sigmoidoscope. A Venturi-type adapter that is connected to the water faucet can be used to provide the suction. A dependable and powerful suction apparatus is a must, especially if bleeding is present or anticipated; bleeding often occurs in rectal punch biopsies. Sigmoidoscopes vary in size, but the usual length is 25 cm. Insertion to the full extent is considered necessary for an adequate examination.

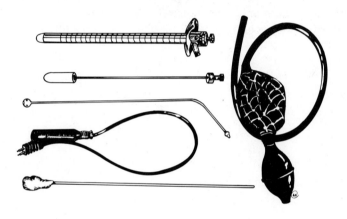

Commonly used equipment for diagnosis and therapy includes the following: a jawed-tooth biopsy forceps, which comes in a variety of sizes and configurations; a cautery snare, which can be placed around the neck of pedunculated lesions; and a ball-tipped cautery, which is used to coagulate bleeding points. The exact settings of the electrocautery equipment vary with the instruments available and should be checked at the time of use.

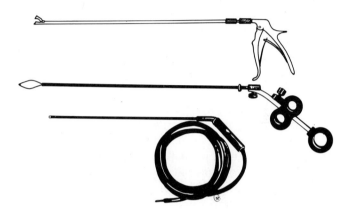

One or several enemas will be required 30 minutes to 1 hour prior to examination in order to empty the lower rectum properly. When colitis or other severe inflammatory diseases of the bowel are suspected, enemas must be used with discrimination.

An assistant is valuable in aiding with sigmoidoscopy. The dominant hand of the operator controls the insufflator, suction, forceps, and electrocautery, while the nondominant hand positions the sigmoidoscope.

Several positions are suitable for sigmoidoscopy, as well as for anoscopy and digital rectal examinations. The patient may be placed in the lateral decubitus position with the knees and hips flexed and the buttocks extended 6 to 8 inches over the edge of the table (A). Manipulation of the sigmoidoscope at the time of withdrawal will be easier if the buttocks extend beyond the table edge. The knee-chest position will usually suffice, since it tends to straighten the rectosigmoid colon by displacing it away from the pelvis (B). The patient kneels with the hips flexed and rests the chest primarily on one shoulder, with the head turned to the opposite side. The arms may be folded underneath the body, or the hands may grip the sides of the table. This position is more difficult for the patient to maintain than the lateral decubitus position.

Special tables are available that flex at the hip area and have attachments to support the head and knees; such a table is probably most comfortable for the patient. It can usually be tipped so that the abdominal contents fall away from the pelvis. The patient usually grips the headrest with both hands and turns the head to one side (C). Proper draping exposes only the anal area.

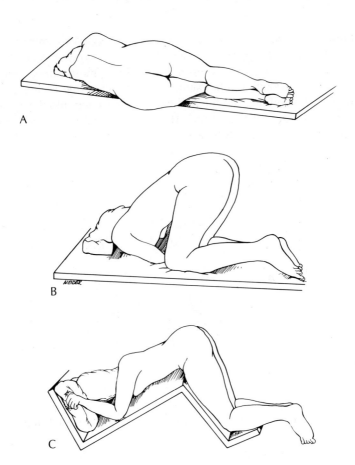

A

B

C

Prior to insertion of the sigmoidoscope, a digital examination should always be made to be sure that there is no obstruction or stricture. The obturator is inserted into the sigmoidoscope, and the tip is thoroughly lubricated. The sigmoidoscope is directed toward the umbilicus in the midline and is inserted into the anus with gentle but firm pressure. The patient should be reassured throughout the procedure, and each step should be explained.

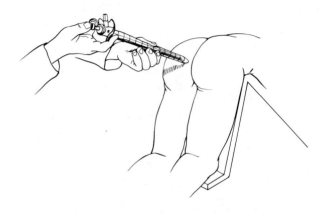

When the sigmoidoscope has been placed 4 cm into the anal canal, the obturator is removed, the anal mucosa visualized through the instrument, and all fluid removed by suctioning.

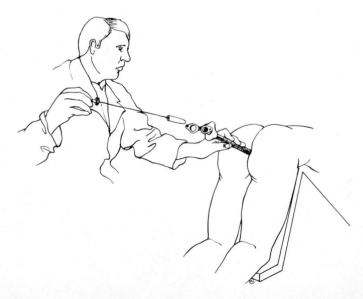

After removal of the obturator, the glass covering is secured over the end of the sigmoidoscope, the insufflator and light sources are attached, and the sigmoidoscope is advanced. Injection of air dilates the rectal lumen, which facilitates identification of structures and helps manipulate the sigmoidoscope into various positions so that it can be advanced.

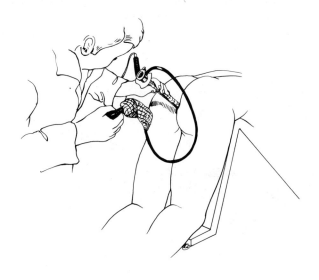

After passing the anal canal and on entering the rectum, the sigmoidoscope is directed posteriorly in the midline toward the hollow of the sacrum. This requires depression of the external portion of the instrument down toward the patient's knees. As the instrument is advanced, it is essential that the lumen be identified at all times to prevent rectal trauma and perforation. Air is gently insufflated as necessary to identify the lumen. If the patient becomes uncomfortable, the glass shield is removed to permit exodus of air under pressure. Continuous suctioning and wiping with swabs will keep the colon free of fluid and feces.

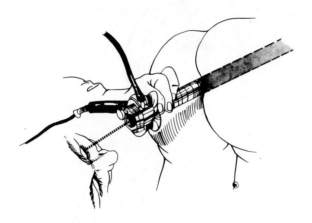

During initial insertion the sigmoidoscope is directed anteriorly as it passes into the anal canal (A). It is then directed posteriorly to conform to the posterior convexity of the rectum (B) and is kept in the midline because this is the position of the rectum. As the rectosigmoid junction is encountered at 14 to 16 cm from the anus, the tip of the instrument is pressed anteriorly and is directed toward the left side because the rectosigmoid curves to the left (C). It is at this point that severe angulation may be present and difficulty in passage of the instrument encountered. If the patient has diverticulitis, it is often impossible to pass the sigmoidoscope further than 15 cm because of pain. Tumors, strictures, and extrinsic masses can obstruct the lumen at any point. In some patients, acute angulation of the rectosigmoid juncture is so extreme that no amount of manipulation will be successful.

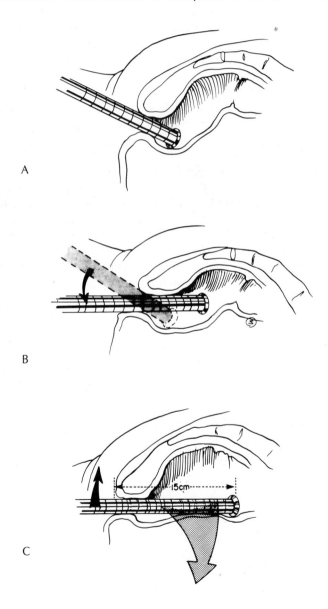

A

B

C

When the sigmoid colon is entered, it can be identified by transverse folds; the rectum has a smooth mucosal surface. Forceful passage should never be attempted. The patient must be reassured that the procedure is proceeding satisfactorily, especially when the rectosigmoid juncture is encountered.

When the sigmoidoscope has been inserted to the maximal extent, the glass covering is removed, and fluid and feces are suctioned or wiped away. After the glass window is replaced, enough air is insufflated to separate the bowel walls, so that the lumen may be clearly visualized. It is at the time of sigmoidoscope withdrawal that careful inspection is performed. Prior to this time the operator is primarily concerned with insertion of the instrument rather than with meticulous examination of the lumen.

During withdrawal, the sigmoidoscope is rotated continuously through a 360° field, so that all surfaces can be seen. Gentle insufflation of air is maintained. The operator may be required to position himself awkwardly so that a complete and thorough examination can be done. As the anorectal juncture is approached, particular care is required for adequate visualization of the posterior rectal wall. When the pectinate line is identified, the instrument is slowly withdrawn, so that the anal canal may be inspected.

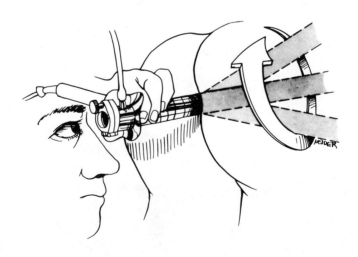

Rectosigmoid disease includes inflammation, ulceration, polyps, tumors, strictures, and perforations, with omentum or perirectal fat protruding. Lesions peculiar to the anus must also be identified. Bleeding points or passage of blood from above should be noted. With severe bleeding, suctioning may not be adequate and a proper examination impossible.

Rectal Biopsy

Some rectal tumors can be adequately excised or "biopsied" in the emergency department. It must be emphasized, however, that lesions more than 10 cm from the anus lie within the intraperitoneal portion of the rectum, and biopsy or excision carries the risk of bowel perforation into the free peritoneal cavity. Excision of all lesions more than 10 cm should therefore be performed in the operating room, after preparation of the bowel. Pedunculated lesions can be removed by applying a snare electrocautery instrument over the lesion, thus dividing and coagulating the base.

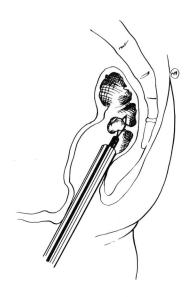

The bowel wall is not tented, since this might result in perforation.

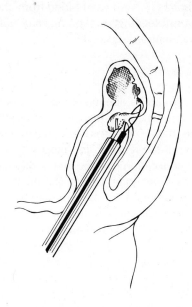

After polyp removal, careful inspection for bleeding is essential. Excellent suction apparatus must be available. Coagulation with a ball-tipped cautery is often required. An electrocoagulating suction apparatus is very helpful in controlling bleeding after biopsy. Rest and avoidance of bowel movements for 24 hours is recommended.

With large, fungating tumors, superficial biopsies with jawed forceps are usually safe at any level. With minimally elevated lesions, the chances of bowel perforation increase, and care must be exercised. Biopsies in the central necrotic portion of ulcerated tumors should be avoided; rather, biopsy specimens should be taken at the edge, where viable tissue can result in a definitive histologic diagnosis. Following biopsy of anything other than large, fungating tumors, barium enemas should be avoided for 5 days. Fulguration and scraping of large superficial lesions are not recommended emergency department procedures; they usually require specialist consultation and hospitalization of the patient. All specimens must be submitted for histologic examination. Cauterization of small lesions without histologic examination should be avoided because a malignant tumor may be missed.

Hemorrhoids

Hemorrhoids are internal or external, depending on whether they originate above or below the pectinate line respectively. External hemorrhoids usually do not cause symptoms until they become thrombosed.

INTERNAL HEMORRHOIDS

Internal hemorrhoids can be diagnosed by palpation when the patient strains or by examination during anoscopy. Prolapse, either partial or complete, is associated with bleeding (particularly during defecation), moisture around the anus, edema, and tenesmus. The treatment of internal hemorrhoids usually requires surgical excision and suturing of the rectal and anal mucosa as an inpatient procedure.

Ligation

The rubber-band ligation technique is available for uncomplicated, well-defined internal hemorrhoids. After gentle dilation of
the anus and insertion of a large anoscope, the internal hemorrhoid is identified. Local or general anesthesia is usually not
necessary. Rubber bands are rolled onto the metal applicator
over a tapered obturator tip that is temporarily attached for this
purpose (A). After the rubber bands have been loaded, the obturator is unscrewed and removed. An Allis clamp is inserted
through the ring of the metal applicator, and the hemorrhoid is
grasped. The applicator is advanced over the hemorrhoid to its
base (B) and the applicator handle is then squeezed, which
forces the stretched rubber ring onto the base of the hemorrhoid
(C). There it strangulates the tissue (D). The hemorrhoid becomes
distended and purple, and after 1 week it sloughs, and the rubber
band is passed from the anus.

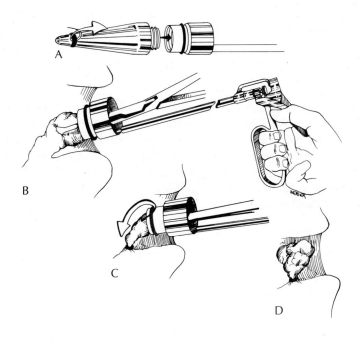

It is not advisable to ligate more than one hemorrhoid at a time. Multiple applications may be necessary. Provided that the ligating point is above the pectinate line, significant pain should not occur. Severe discomfort indicates that the anal canal mucosa is caught in the rubber band, which should be removed. Bleeding is not usually a significant problem.

Injection

Injection treatment is suitable for most smaller hemorrhoids. Larger hemorrhoids that remain prolapsed after defecation and require digital replacement are less effectively treated by the injection technique. Contraindications to this mode of therapy include the following: (1) external piles or skin-covered components (injection is painful because of the cutaneous innervation of the distal third of the anal canal); (2) thrombosed hemorrhoids; (3) pregnancy; and (4) associated anal lesions.

A solution of phenol in almond oil is used for injection. Necessary equipment includes a large-diameter proctoscope 2¾ inches long, a 10-ml Luer-Lok controlled syringe, and a 3-inch needle that is either straight or slightly angulated. Special preparation of the bowel is usually not necessary.

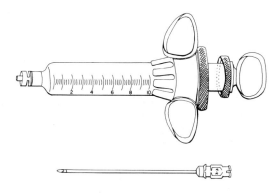

With the patient in the lithotomy position, the anoscope is introduced, and the anorectal ring is identified by the projection of the puborectalis posteriorly. The circumferential position of the ring can then be estimated. This ring lies above the superior aspect of the hemorrhoid and is the site of injection for each hemorrhoid. The hemorrhoid itself is *not* injected.

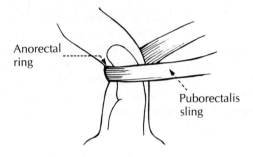

The anoscope must be manipulated and angled to obtain the proper position to permit injection above each of the three main hemorrhoid groups.

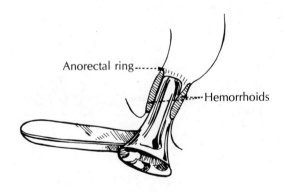

With the anoscope positioned just proximal to the anorectal ring and yet above the internal hemorrhoid, the needle is introduced under the mucosa with a quick jabbing movement. It must usually then be withdrawn slightly to place the needle tip submucosally. Injection of 5 ml of solution then begins. Initially, small amounts should be injected to ensure proper localization of the needle tip. If there is resistance to injection, the needle is probably too deeply positioned and should be pulled back slightly. If a hard, white induration of the mucosa supervenes, the fluid is being injected too superficially into the mucosa. Proper injection produces a diffuse, ballooned, edematous wheal. For each hemorrhoid, 5 ml is injected, using a total of 15 ml for most patients. No special care is needed after injection. However, the patient should be told to avoid strenuous activities and bowel movements for 12 to 24 hours.

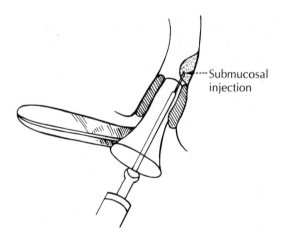

Submucosal injection

Some discomfort, often described as an aching in the anal canal, is experienced by a majority of patients during the injection. Severe pain indicates that the injection has been given too low in the anal canal in the area of somatic innervation.

Injection treatment invokes a fibrous reaction in the submucosa that constricts the arteries and veins associated with the hemorrhoid. Injection treatment is most effective for bleeding hemorrhoids, less so for large, fibrosed, and freely prolapsing hemorrhoids.

The most common complications are necrosis and injection ulcers that usually heal spontaneously. Rarely, submucosal abscess, rectal bleeding, prostatic abscess, temporary rectal stricture, and granulomatous lesions have been observed. Fatalities from this procedure are essentially unknown.

THROMBOSED EXTERNAL HEMORRHOIDS

Although external hemorrhoids are usually asymptomatic; when they become thrombosed and filled with clot, exquisite pain occurs, and the patient seeks immediate relief. Early, minimally distended thrombosed hemorrhoids may be treated conservatively with sitz baths, local analgesics, and stool softeners. An acutely thrombosed hemorrhoid should be incised.

With the patient in the lateral decubitus or lithotomy position, the anal area is exposed. Shaving is usually not required. The area is prepared with antiseptic solution. The area surrounding the thrombosed hemorrhoid is injected with a local anesthetic, avoiding injection into the thrombosed hemorrhoid, since this would cause further distention and increase pain. A radial incision is made through the extent of the distended mucosa (A), and the thrombus is extruded (B). Mild to moderate bleeding may be encountered, but it can be controlled by pressure. After removal of the thrombus, the skin edges shrivel and fold together (C). Suture closure is not required.

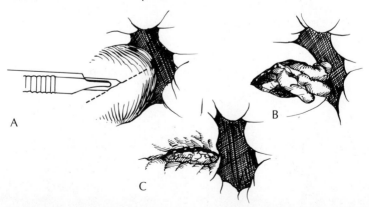

Postoperatively, the patient is treated with oral analgesics, sitz baths, and stool softeners. A complete anal and rectal examination should be done a week later, when symptoms have resolved.

Perirectal Abscess

There are several types of perirectal abscesses. Treatment of those above the levator ani muscle (pelvirectal or supralevator) requires hospitalization and general anesthesia. Similarly, deep-seated ischiorectal abscesses should not be drained in the emergency department. The more superficial abscess (perianal), either those in a submucosal position or those lying somewhat deeper but having an obviously "pointing area" in the skin, may be incised and drained under local anesthesia on an outpatient basis. To locate an abscess, it may be necessary to perform needle aspiration to detect pus (differentiation from diffuse cellulitis) and to determine exactly where the incision should be made. The rectum is examined prior to incision and drainage; however, because of exquisite tenderness, this may be difficult.

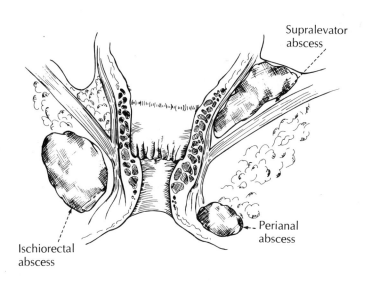

Supralevator abscess

Perianal abscess

Ischiorectal abscess

After localization of the abscess and infiltration of anesthesia (A), a radial incision is made in a limited fashion until pus is obtained (B). An opening large enough to admit a finger is completed, and the abscess cavity is then explored with the digit to identify in which direction the incision should be enlarged (C). The abscess is widely opened and pus evacuated. If the patient shows evidence of sepsis, antibiotics should be started. Otherwise, in the absence of systemic symptoms, incision and drainage alone will suffice. Often, the abscess originates from the anal crypts, and a communication with the pectinate line may be identified. In most cases, one must be satisfied with drainage of the abscess only, since exploration of the anus is too painful to be permitted by the patient. Sitz baths, meticulous cleansing, heat, and stool softeners constitute the usual medical treatment following operation.

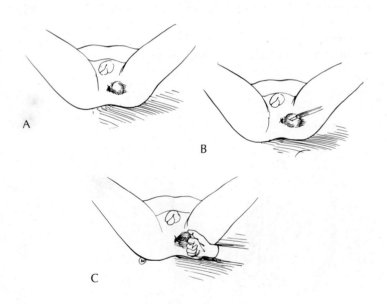

A

B

C

Fecal Impaction

Fecal impaction typically occurs in elderly, bedridden patients with reduced bowel motility. Impaction may be the result of a pathologic condition causing partial obstruction, dehydration or improper diet, or may not have an obvious cause. Patients can present with constipation or diarrhea. For this reason it is essential that all patients with any type of bowel complaint have a rectal examination. This is especially true of patients who are older, particularly those in nursing homes.

The diagnosis is easily made once the finger is inserted into the rectum. Hard, inspissated fecal material is easily palpated. If the mass is not solidified, enemas may permit passage of stool. Oil retention enemas are required if the mass is firm and fixed. Mineral oil (200 ml) is inserted and retained for at least 1 or 2 hours. This is followed with saline enemas and repeated rectal examinations. On occasion, the hard feces must be manually broken up and then treated with oil retention and saline enemas. These steps should be repeated as necessary. Possible causes should be searched for once the patient has recovered.

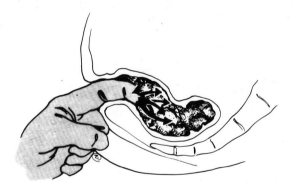

Condyloma Acuminatum
Condylomata occur frequently in the perianal area and are treated in the same manner as is described in Chapter 12.

Anal Fissure
Anal fissures typically occur in the posterior midline in females. These lacerations of the anal mucosa are usually caused by constipation and hard stools. A hypertrophied skin tag may be seen at the external edge of the fissure. A variety of lesions can mimic anal fissures.

Most superficial fissures will heal with topical anesthetics, sitz baths, careful cleansing of the anus, and stool softeners. Operative excision on an inpatient basis is occasionally indicated when conservative measures fail.

14

Procedures on the Upper and Lower Extremities

Marshall B. Conrad

Many patients who arrive in an emergency department following a trauma will have suffered bony injuries in addition to other problems. By and large, the management of fractures or dislocations should be left to the care of physicians especially trained to deal with such problems. Similarly, the handling of trauma or infections of the hand should be reserved for surgeons who by virtue of their training and experience can expect to obtain the maximal return of function. It is the intent of this chapter to outline the examinations necessary to detect disease or injury of the bones and joints, as well as the procedures that should be performed by the personnel of the emergency and outpatient departments.

Interpretation of roentgenograms is a skill that can be learned only by daily exposure to a large volume of both normal and abnormal films, with review under the guidance of a trained radiologist. This skill is mandatory, however, for all those who manage acutely ill or injured persons.

All persons who arrive at a hospital following a major trauma should have been properly splinted, as is outlined in Chapter 1. It is not inappropriate to make the plea that any patient who presents with even minimal signs of significant bony or soft tissue injury can be made more comfortable by a properly applied splint, or bandage, or both. Remember that it is most important to evaluate the condition of the circulation distal to the level of injury in an extremity. If the circulation is adequate, indicated by the presence of pulses and the capillary return of the nail beds, these findings must be reevaluated and documented after a splint or bandage is applied.

Similarly, the function of the major nerves must be tested both before and after splints are applied. *The functions of the major peripheral nerves that may be lost following injury include the following:*

1. Axillary: Abduction of the upper arm at the shoulder.
2. Musculocutaneous: Flexion of the elbow.
3. Radial: Dorsiflexion of the hand at the wrist.
4. Median: Opposition of the thumb.
5. Ulnar: Spreading and closing of the fingers.
6. Femoral: Extension of the leg at the knee.
7. Tibial: Plantar flexion of the foot.
8. Peroneal: Dorsiflexion of the foot.

The physician experienced in the primary care of acutely ill or injured persons learns to perform the preliminary evaluation in an orderly, routine manner, to avoid the pitfall of a missed lesion because the area was not surveyed.

Closed Fractures

At all times, keep in mind the dictum "Do no harm." For this reason it is essential that the initial examination for closed fractures be made while the patient is still on the stretcher on which he or she arrived. This is not to say that an ambulance with its crew should be out of service for the hours necessary to do a complete roentgenographic survey or while minor wounds are treated. However, it is most important that the patient not be subjected to hurried, rough handling. In like fashion, a patient who presents with an obvious deformity or swelling of an arm or leg need not be subjected to the pain elicited by moving the fracture site just to demonstrate crepitus of the bone ends or the presence of abnormal motion.

The diagnosis and initial care of injuries to the skull and vertebral column are considered elsewhere in this text. It is emphasized again, however, that immobilization of the vertebral column for a suspected injury must take precedence over any other bony injury, open or closed, and is exceeded in importance only by the need to maintain a patent airway, ventilation, and circulation of the blood to the vital organs.

Open Fractures

The hemorrhage from any open wound with or without a fracture must be controlled by the application of sterile dry gauze well padded using multilayered gauze dressings, held in place by a conforming gauze bandage.

Shock must be combated by positioning the patient in a slight Trendelenburg position on a long backboard. The administration of intravenous fluids is mandatory. If a fracture is apparent at the wound site, the extremity is handled with mild traction while the bandage and then the splint are applied. There should be no attempt to reduce the bone ends back under the skin, but if the extremity is badly crushed, the greatest attention should be paid to placing the distal parts in the position that allows for the best circulation, whether or not this means that the ends are retracted. If such an extremity is to be salvaged, there will need to be very extensive debridement and irrigation of the wounds, including reexposing the fracture site after the patient has arrived in the operating suite. The strong injunction promulgated by less informed physicians against ever retracting bone ends under the skin is based on a lack of understanding of all the problems that may be involved.

Shoulder Girdle

After the examination of the head and back, including palpation of the facial bones, has ruled out problems in these areas, the bones of the shoulder girdle should be examined, including the clavicle, scapula, and proximal humerus.

CLAVICLE

Ordinarily, the clavicle can be palpated throughout its length and can be visually compared with the opposite side. Tenderness or swelling over the injured side suggests a hematoma from a fracture site. Since the clavicle acts as a strut in supporting the shoulder joint, it is readily apparent that any motion of this joint will produce pain at the fracture site. As a consequence, the conscious patient will attempt to splint the arm by supporting the injured side with the uninjured extremity.

Fractures of the body of the clavicle are customarily splinted by a figure-eight bandage, using elastic bandage or triangular bandages.

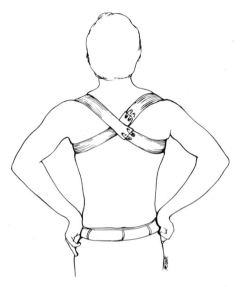

In either case the anterior surface of the axilla as well as the back of the neck should be well padded to avoid discomfort to the patient.

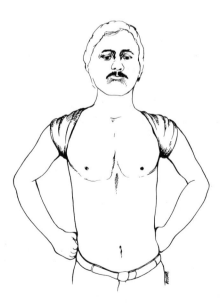

Commercial versions with Velcro fastening are quickly applied and easily adjusted.

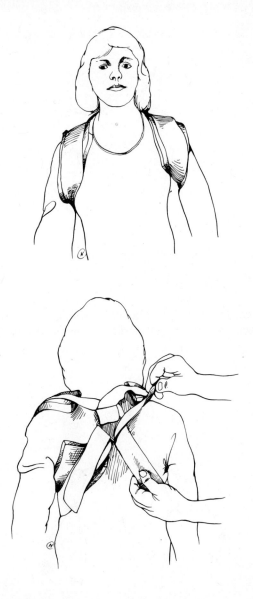

In the adult, supporting the weight of the arm with an arm sling may reduce the pain. Similarly, binding the arm to the chest wall with a Velpeau bandage will combat the downward sagging at the fracture site.

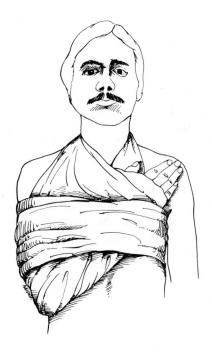

STERNOCLAVICULAR AND ACROMIOCLAVICAL JOINTS
Injuries of the articulations of the clavicle are painful on motion of the affected joint. Not infrequently, the dislocated bone presents by the prominence of one end of the clavicle as compared with the same end of the opposite clavicle. As with other fractures or dislocations, roentgenograms are essential in confirming the clinical impression.

Anterior Sternoclavicular Dislocations
The anteriorly dislocated clavicle is apparent by the prominence of the sternal end and is most readily reduced by having the patient lie supine and then pushing the patient's shoulder upward, outward, and backward with one hand and pushing the proximal clavicle back into its normal position. The arm is then supported in a sling.

Posterior Sternoclavicular Dislocations
A posterior dislocation of the medial end of the clavicle is apparent by the loss of contour of the sternoclavicular joint area. If such a dislocation is suspected, detailed roentgenographic views of the posterior sternum must be ordered. The end of the clavicle can push on the trachea or esophagus; to avoid these complications, this type of dislocation must be reduced, which usually requires an operative procedure.

Idiopathic enlargement of the sternoclavicular joint may occur and may be confused with a dislocation of the medial end of the clavicle. However, it is without clinical significance. Dislocation is ruled out by roentgenograms that reveal the enlarged joint but with normal alignment of the apposing bones.

Acromioclavicular Dislocations

The dislocation of the acromioclavicular joint is judged to be *incomplete* if the coracoclavicular ligament (trapazoid and conoid components) is partially intact (A), *complete* if this ligament has been torn apart (B).

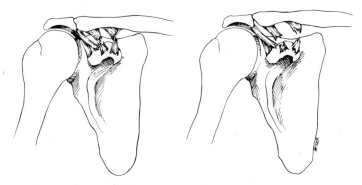

Ruptured trapezoid lig.   Ruptured trapezoid lig. and conoid lig.

The incomplete dislocation may be managed with a sling that supports the humerus upward. If the dislocation is complete, open reduction and repair is the treatment of choice.

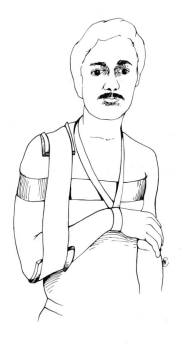

SCAPULA

Fractures of the body of the scapula are uncommon, since the bone is protected on both the anterior and posterior surfaces by muscle.

Swelling in the area of the body of the scapula following direct trauma is most commonly due to hematoma formation in the area, but a fracture must be ruled out by anteroposterior and tangential x-ray views of the scapula, especially when severe trauma has been inflicted on that part of the chest wall.

The treatment of fractures or other severe trauma to the area consists of supporting the arm of the affected side in a sling and swath.

ACROMION

Fractures of the acromion usually result from direct trauma to the area. The treatment is to support the arm in a sling and swath.

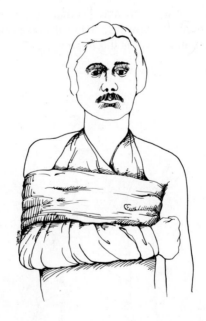

SURGICAL NECK OF THE HUMERUS AND GLENOID CAVITY

Fractures of the surgical neck of the humerus and glenoid cavity usually follow falls on the outstretched arm. The diagnosis is confirmed by roentgenograms of the area.

The treatment is to support the arm of that side with a sling while encouraging motion; early motion is most important in the elderly. To achieve an accurate reduction, fractures of the glenoid or neck of the humerus in young people with displacement may require traction or open reduction after the patient has been hospitalized.

DISLOCATION OF THE SHOULDER

Dislocation of the shoulder is the most common dislocation in humans, constituting almost 50 percent of all dislocations. The usual cause is a fall on an outstretched hand, which forces the head of the humerus beneath the coracoid process. The next

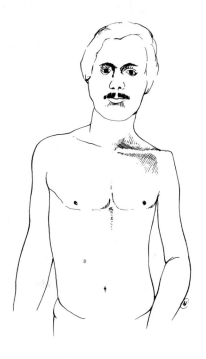

most common dislocation is for the head to be forced beneath the glenoid fossa. The diagnosis is usually apparent, for the normal curved appearance of the deltoid area is flattened, and the distance between the acromion and the point of the elbow is lengthened. Roentgenograms are required to rule out fractures of the clavicle or upper end of the humerus and to confirm the diagnosis. The neurologic and vascular status should be checked before x-rays are made or reduction is attempted.

The simplest, most effective method of reducing glenohumeral dislocations is to lay the patient face down on a stretcher with the dislocated arm hanging over the side. Then a bucket is strapped to the patient's hand and filled with water. If there are no contraindications, the patient also may be given 5 mg of diazepam (Valium) intravenously to aid in muscle relaxation. This should allow the humerus to reduce itself.

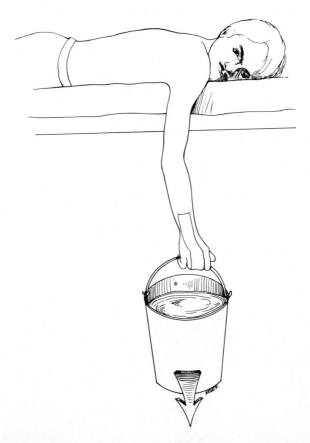

Lateral traction on the humerus coupled with rotation of the arm may be necessary to assist the head of the humerus back into the glenoid fossa. After the dislocation has been reduced, the arm should be supported by a sling and swath. Recurrent dislocations will require operative intravention to repair the tear of the muscles around the glenoid fossa.

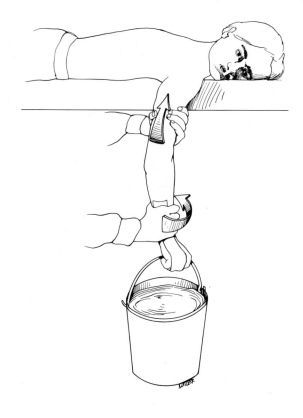

HUMERUS

Impacted fractures of the proximal humerus should be immobilized in a Velpeau dressing or a sling and swath. A hanging cast is considered by some to be the treatment of choice for fractures of the shaft of the humerus, although other physicians prefer other methods of management. Approximately 5 days after the hanging cast is applied, roentgenograms should be repeated. If the position is unsatisfactory, the cast must be adjusted. Open reduction and internal fixation may be necessary. Patients with open fractures or with neurologic or vascular deficits should be admitted to the hospital for management by open reduction.

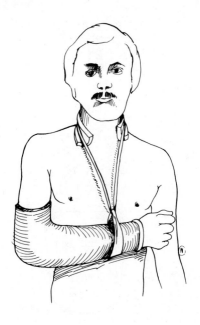

Elbow Joint

Patients with fractures and dislocations of the elbow area must be admitted to the hospital for manipulation and reduction, either closed or open. Because of the possibility of vascular or neurologic deficits, these injuries must be considered surgical emergencies.

Injuries of the proximal radius and ulna, unless the bone is undisplaced, must be managed after the patient's admission to the hospital for reduction under general anesthesia.

Undisplaced fractures may be managed by a posterior plaster splint from the hand to the shoulder. The splinted extremity should be supported by a sling, and the patient should be referred to an orthopedic surgeon.

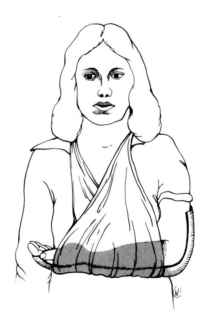

Colles' Fracture of the Wrist

Colles' fracture of the wrist is very common in the aging population and often follows falls on the outstretched arm. The distal fragments are displaced dorsally. This results in the typical "silver-fork" deformity diagnostic of the injury.

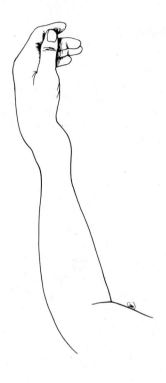

Colles' fractures of the wrist are not surgical emergencies, but the sooner they are reduced, the greater the comfort for the patient. The quickest method of obtaining anesthesia is to introduce 10 ml of 1% lidocaine into the hematoma of the fracture site under sterile conditions.

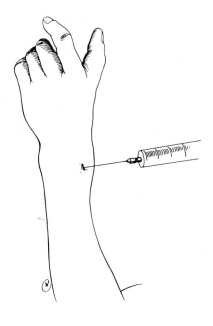

Traction on the site can be obtained with "finger traps" coupled with weight on the upper arm to distract the fracture.

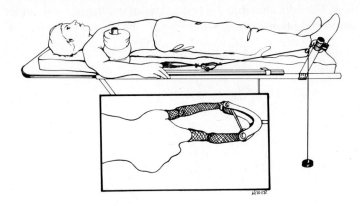

After the muscle spasm has been overcome, pressure is exerted over the distal radial fragment to correct the deformity and thereby restore the normal angle of the wrist joint.

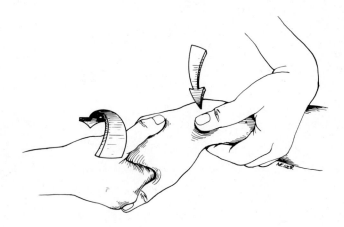

The position can be held by placing the hand in ulnar deviation with slight flexion of the hand on the wrist. The cast should include the forearm pronated on the upper arm, with the elbow held at 90° flexion. A postreduction roentgenogram must be made to confirm that the reduction has been maintained while the cast was applied.

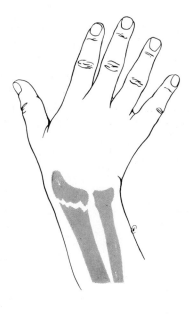

Carpal Bones

The most common injuries of the carpal bones are fracture of the navicular bone and dislocation of the lunate bone. These injuries most often result from falls on the outstretched hand and can be difficult to diagnose unless a high index of suspicion exists on the part of the examining physician.

FRACTURE OF THE NAVICULAR BONE
The patient usually complains of pain on motion of the wrist, and swelling of the area is present. Maximal tenderness is elicited by pressure on the anatomic snuff box. The diagnosis is confirmed by special oblique views of the wrist in addition to the customary anteroposterior and lateral roentgenograms. Even if a navicular fracture is not visualized in a symptomatic patient, immobilization for 10 days in a cast that should include the thumb, followed by repeat x-ray studies, should rule out a fractured navicular bone. If no fracture is present, no harm has been done by the cast.

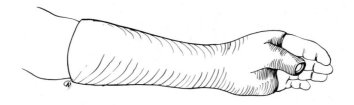

DISLOCATION OF THE LUNATE BONE
In dislocation of the lunate bone, the patient presents with a history of a fall on the hand, severe pain, and limited motion of the wrist joint. The lateral roentgenogram will reveal that the lunate bone is not articulating with the capitate.

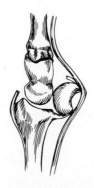

An attempt may be made to reduce the dislocation under regional block anesthesia. The patient's elbow is flexed, and one assistant provides countertraction on the upper arm. Another assistant provides strong traction on the patient's hand, with ulnar deviation (A). The surgeon applies pressure on the dislocated bone with his thumbs at the same time as the hand is hyperextended (B). When the lunate bone is reduced, the wrist will again have its normal range of motion (C, D). The hand is held in neutral position with a plaster cast extended to the distal ends of the metacarpals. Open reduction of the dislocation may be necessary. Fractures of the carpal bones, if undisplaced, may be treated by a cast from the elbow to the proximal interphalangeal joints.

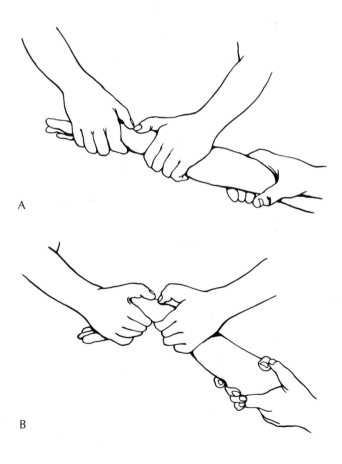

A

B

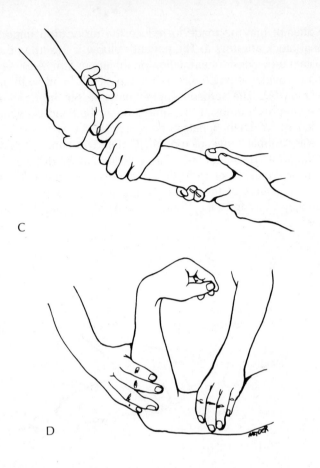

C

D

FRACTURES AND DISLOCATIONS OF
THE METACARPALS AND PHALANGES

Fractures of the first and second metacarpals are difficult to manage and most probably will require accurate reduction and sometimes internal flexation. Undisplaced fractures of the metacarpals
may be immobilized in a cast from the elbow to the proximal
interphalangeal joints. Dislocations of the metacarpophalangeal
joints are reduced by traction in the axis of the metacarpal under
local anesthesia, obtained by infiltrating the area with 1%
lidocaine.

A dislocated first metacarpal is reduced by manual traction. Pressure is applied to the joint under traction. After reduction, the forearm and hand are held with a short cast.

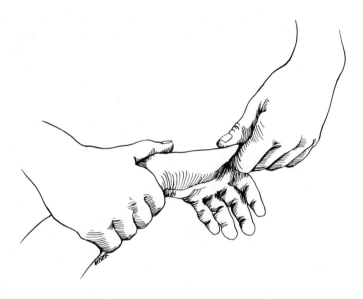

A fracture of the distal metacarpal is managed by infiltrating the site with 1% lidocaine. Then, a well-padded cast is applied that incorporates the involved finger and those adjacent to it. The surgeon applies pressure over the distal fragment to mold the cast and reduce the fracture. All casts involving the fingers must hold the various joints in slight flexion.

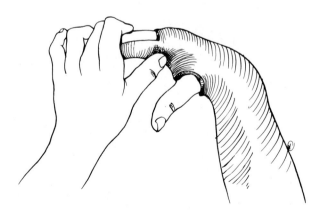

Phalanges

A dislocation of one of the phalanges is usually easily reduced by traction with or without local anesthesia.

A fracture of the base of the proximal phalanx in children (Salter type II) (A) is difficult to reduce unless a pencil is inserted between the fractured and the adjacent finger, and the fingers are squeezed together to force the base back into its normal relationship (B).

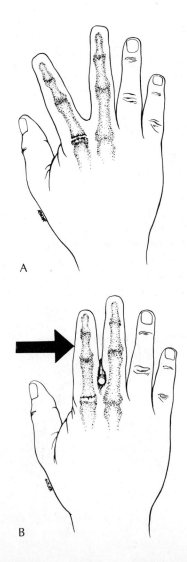

A

B

Baseball Finger

The extensor tendon may rupture or its insertion on the distal phalanx may be avulsed following a blow to the extended finger, as might occur when a fly ball is caught on the fingertips—hence the name. Roentgenograms are mandatory to rule out a fracture.

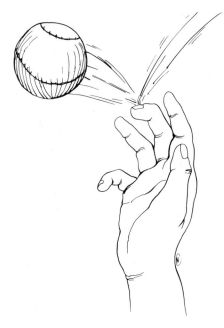

A wide variety of treatments have been advocated for baseball finger, but satisfactory healing will usually result if immobilization is maintained long enough, i.e., 6 to 8 weeks. If the patient is seen soon after the injury, the finger is held with an aluminum finger splint applied over the dorsum of the finger to hold the distal interphalangeal joint in hyperextension and the middle and proximal phalanges flexed.

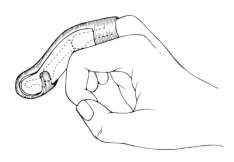

Lower Extremities

Patients with most fractures and dislocations of the pelvis, hip joint, femur, and knee joint should be admitted to the hospital for management, except under certain circumstances.

KNEE

Dislocated Patella

Dislocation of the patella is usually reduced by placing the knee joint in full extension. Pressure with the thumbs, with or without anesthesia, should reduce the bone. If this does not occur, the patient must be admitted to the hospital for reduction, open or closed, under general anesthesia.

Because of the valgus angle of the female knee, patellar injuries are more common in females than in males. Chondromalacia is also more common in the female.

After reduction has been achieved, the knee joint, if it is distended, may be aspirated under sterile conditions and a plaster cylinder applied.

Examination of the Knee Joint

Spasm of the hamstring muscles induced by injury to a knee cartilage prevents complete extension of the joint, just as an effusion in the knee joint also prevents complete extension. Absence of a joint effusion tends to exclude a tear of a cruciate ligament or collateral ligament. Therefore, if the knee joint can be extended completely, serious injury to one of the cartilages or ligaments is unlikely.

Injuries of the ligaments of the knee joint commonly follow blows to the side of the extended joint, i.e., being "clipped" from the side. A semilunar cartilage is most frequently torn when the joint is rotated while the foot and leg are fixed, as when a football player carrying the ball twists to avoid a tackler when his cleats are firmly fixed in the turf.

Patients with these injuries usually present with a painful swollen joint, and if a cartilage has been torn and lies in between the femur and tibia, the joint may be locked in some degree of flexion. Pressure over the affected cartilage elicits pain.

A badly swollen joint requires aspiration and may require that the patient be admitted to the hospital for bed rest. The subsequent management may well include surgery.

Collateral Ligaments

Tears of the medial and lateral ligaments are frequently demonstrated by the abnormal opening of the joint on the affected side. Sometimes the diagnosis requires an examination under anesthesia. The range of medial and lateral motion produced by the examiner is negligible in a normal knee. If the ligaments are torn, a movement of 10° to 15° may be produced.

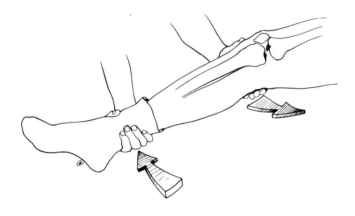

Cruciate Ligaments

ANTERIOR. The anterior cruciate ligament is tense when the knee joint is fully extended. If the anterior ligament has been torn, the tibia can be moved anteriorly on the femur.

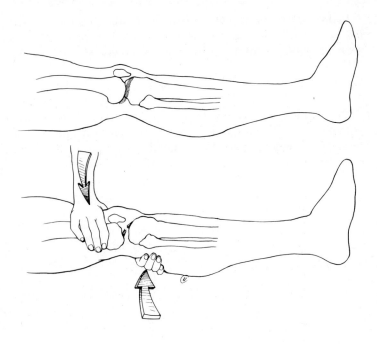

POSTERIOR. When the knee is flexed to 90°, the posterior cruciate ligament is tense. When the patient is sitting with the foot and pelvis fixed, a torn posterior ligament is demonstrated by moving the tibia back on the femur. A fresh tear of a posterior cruciate ligament may present as a hematoma in the popliteal fossa.

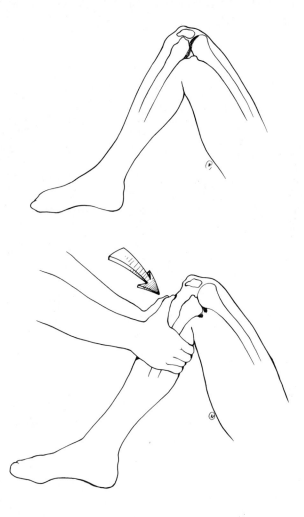

LOWER LEG AND ANKLE

Patients with fractures of the lower leg and ankle should be admitted to the hospital before or after the cast is applied, so that the extremity can be kept elevated on pillows and the toes checked to avoid the problem of vascular compromise from swelling. Pads must be applied over body prominences to avoid necrosis of the skin.

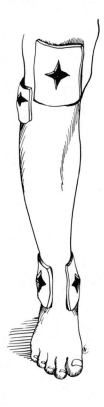
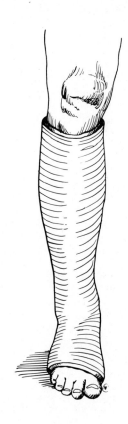

Fracture dislocations of the ankle joint may need immediate reduction and splinting even before roentgenograms are made. The risk of necrosis of the tense skin is great if this dictum is not followed.

FOOT
Dislocations of the metatarsals and phalanges of the toes are usually easily reduced by traction.

Metatarsals
A simple, undisplaced fracture of one of the metatarsals can be treated by an elastic wrap of the foot and lower leg. The patient must use crutches for 2 to 3 weeks to avoid weight bearing. Patients with more extensive fractures of the metatarsals may need to be admitted to the hospital for bed rest, with elevation of the extremity. These patients are then usually treated by application of a cast to the foot and lower leg.

Phalanges
Fractures of the phalanges are easily managed by painting the foot and toes with tincture of benzoin. A gauze pad is placed between the affected toe and its neighbors, and the toes are taped together. Any malalignment is corrected by traction before the taping is done.

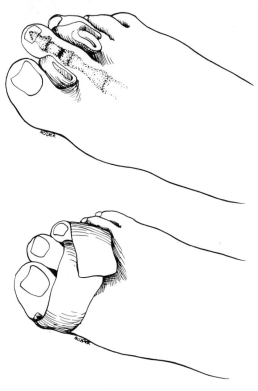

Subungual Hematoma

Fractures of the terminal phalanges that occur when a door is slammed on a finger or toe are usually accompanied by a hematoma under the nail. This is most readily evacuated by burning a hole through the nail with a red-hot paper clip heated in a burner and held with a forceps.

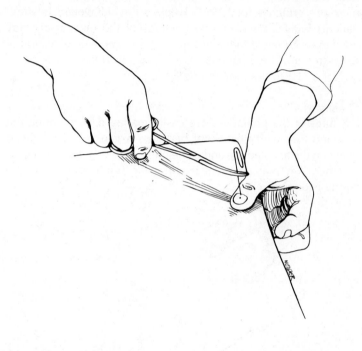

Special Techniques
SKELETAL TRACTION PINS

Customarily, skeletal traction devices are applied after the patient has been admitted to the hospital. At times, however, the pins may be inserted in the emergency department for traction to be applied after admission. The pin must be inserted under sterile conditions, using local anesthesia. The most common sites are through the proximal tibia, keeping distal to the epiphysis, through the distal femur, or through the olecranon.

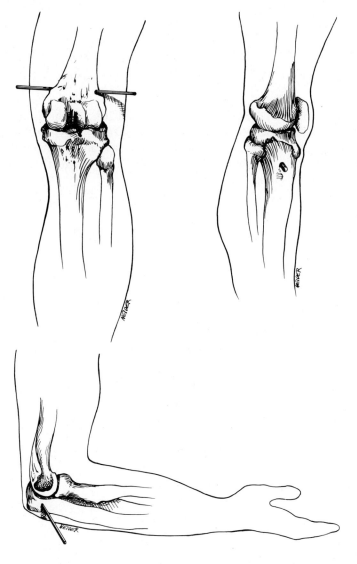

ASPIRATION OF JOINTS

Injection of medications into joints is no longer in vogue in the management of arthritic conditions. Aspiration of joints to evacuate blood or other fluids is done for pain relief or to obtain material to be examined for crystals (gout, pseudogout) or bacteria (septic arthritis).

The skin must be carefully prepared as for any other surgical procedure, and the needle site should be anesthetized with 1 to 2 ml of 1% lidocaine.

Usually, a disposable dry syringe with an 18-gauge needle is used. For the hip joint, an 18-gauge spinal needle may be needed.

Wrist

For aspiration of the wrist the joint is flexed 20°, and the aspirating needle is inserted through the anesthetized skin. The needle and syringe are held perpendicular to the skin and inserted into the joint between the radius and carpal bones, lateral to the flexor pollicis longus tendon.

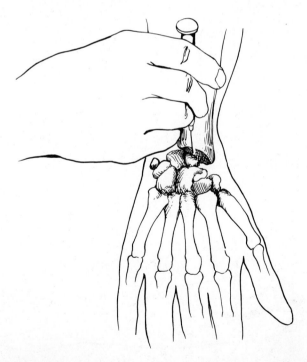

Elbow

For aspiration of the elbow the needle is inserted into the radiohumeral joint just distal to the lateral epicondyle.

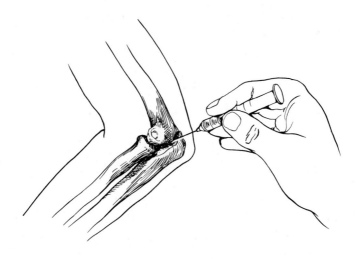

Anterior Approach to the Shoulder Joint

For aspiration of the shoulder joint the patient is positioned sitting upright. The needle is inserted just medial to the humerus and just below the tip of the coracoid process.

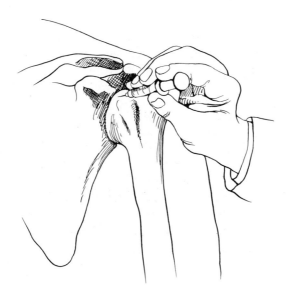

Shoulder Bursa

For aspiration of a shoulder bursa the needle is inserted perpendicular to the skin beneath the acromion.

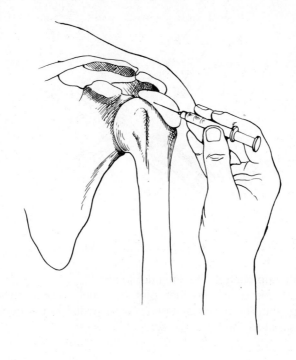

Knee

The knee is aspirated from either the medial or lateral side with the leg extended. The needle is inserted between the patella and femur, beneath the midportion of the patella.

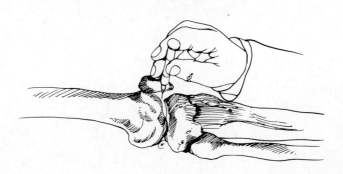

Ankle

The usual site for aspiration of the ankle is between the medial malleolus and the anterior tibial tendon. The needle must be inserted 2 to 3 cm.

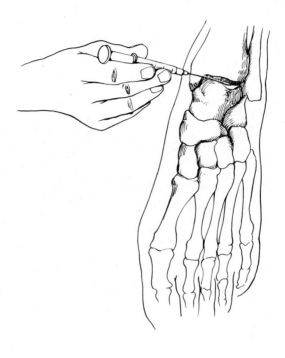

Hip

In the hip, the aspiration site is at a point 2 cm distal to the midpoint on a line drawn between the anterosuperior iliac spine and the pubic spine. The 3-inch needle is inserted slightly posteriorly and slightly medially at a 60° angle to the skin.

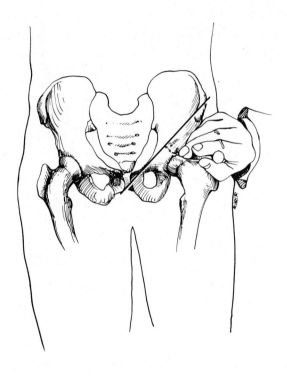

15

Burns

Allen P. Klippel

Burns are without a doubt the most catastrophic illness, financially and physiologically, that may be visited on any patient. Prompt recognition of the severity of the injury and initiation of the most appropriate therapy can do much to ameliorate some of the ravages of burns. Risk of a fatal outcome is twice as great in burns in children under 2 years of age, in adults over 50, and in patients with preexisting severe constitutional disease.

PREHOSPITAL MANAGEMENT

Remove all burned clothing to ensure that no smoldering fabric remains in contact with the patient. Cover the burned areas with a sterile sheet or sterile burn dressing. It is helpful to cool the area with sterile water, or ice bags, or both. If possible, start intravenous fluids, usually Ringer's lactate, even if the trip to the hospital will be brief. Start the fluids only through unburned skin.

ESTIMATION OF BURNED AREA

Estimation of the burned area is necessary for calculation of fluid requirements and to indicate the patients who need to be hospitalized.

Allow 1 percent for full-thickness burns (third-degree) and 0.5 percent for partial-thickness burns when calculating fluid requirements by the usual rules. One-half of the fluid calculated is administered in the first 8 hours and the remainder in the next 16 hours.

FLUID AND ELECTROLYTES
Brooke Formula
FIRST 24 HOURS. The following are administered in the first 24 hours: colloid (plasma, albumin), 0.5 ml/kg body weight/% burn; electrolytes (Ringer's lactate), 1.5 ml/kg body weight/% burn; 5% dextrose in water, 2,000 ml. For children calculate at 160 ml/kg up to age 2, 100 ml/kg for ages 2 to 5, and 80 ml/kg for ages 6 to 8 to determine the amount of 5% dextrose in water to be administered.

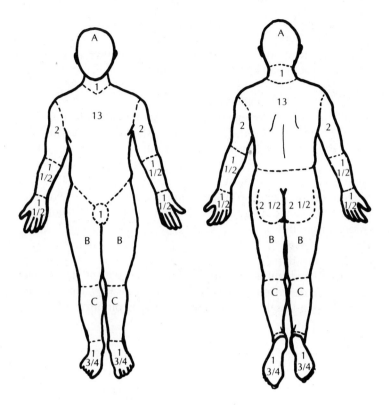

Relative percentage of areas affected by growth

	Age in years					
	0	1	5	10	15	Adult
A. 1/2 of head	9 1/2	8 1/2	6 1/2	5 1/2	4 1/2	3 1/2
B. 1/2 of one thigh	2 3/4	3 1/4	4	4 1/4	4 1/2	4 3/4
C. 1/2 of one leg	2 1/2	2 1/2	2 3/4	3	3 1/4	3 1/2

SECOND 24 HOURS. One-half the calculated volume of colloid and electrolyte solution is administered in the second 24 hours, but the same volume of the glucose in water is given.

Electrolyte Formula
The electrolyte formula should consist of 3 to 4 ml of Ringer's lactate/kg body weight/% burn. Resuscitation with hypertonic solutions has been recommended, but as yet is not generally accepted. With either formula the fluid amounts should result in a urinary volume of 30 to 50 ml per hour.

DEPTH OF BURN

First-Degree Burns

In first-degree burns, only erythema that blanches on pressure is visible. The area is painful to the touch.

Superficial Second-Degree Burns

In superficial second-degree burns, erythema with intact or ruptured blisters is observed. The skin under the blisters is erythematous. The area is usually very tender to the touch.

Deep Second-Degree Burns

In deep second-degree burns, the skin is white, dry, and soft. The area may have reduced sensitivity to touch or pinprick, but sensation is not absent.

Third-Degree Burns

In third-degree burns, the skin is brownish, with a stiff, tough surface. Thrombosed skin vessels may be visible. The area of involved skin usually is insensitive even to a pinprick.

First degree burn

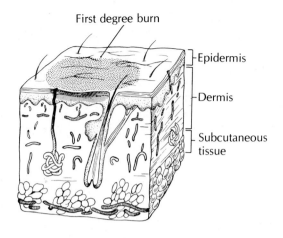

Epidermis

Dermis

Subcutaneous
tissue

Second degree burn (blisters)

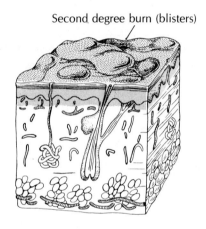

Third degree burn

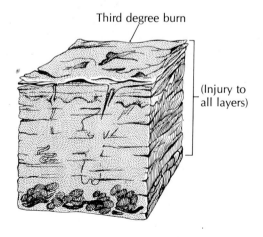

(Injury to
all layers)

PULMONARY PROBLEMS

Only the inhalation of live steam will produce respiratory tract burns. Most pulmonary problems arising from fires result from the inhalation of the toxic products of combustion.

1. Obtain a history of the type of exposure. (Many burning plastics release toxic substances.)
2. Respiratory problems are most likely if the patient was trapped in a room or other closed area.
3. Check for carbon particles in the nose or mouth or for burned nasal hair.
4. Check cough-produced sputum for carbon particles.
5. Draw blood gases, including carbmonoxyhemoglobin, if available.
6. Wheezing on inspiration or expiration may or may not be heard on auscultation, but is a sign of respiratory compromise.
7. Nasotracheal intubation or endotracheal intubation with ventilatory assistance by a volume-cycled respirator is indicated to assist the patient suffering from severe smoke inhalation. Elective tracheostomy should be considered.
8. Methylprednisolone sodium succinate, 15 to 30 mg/kg/24 hr, may be administered for 2 days.
9. Frequent endotracheal suctioning is necessary.

INDICATIONS FOR HOSPITALIZATION

The following patients should be admitted to the hospital:

1. Patients with burns of both hands, both feet, face, neck, or perineum unless the burns are superficial.
2. Patients over 50 years of age or under 2 if more than 10 percent of the body is burned.
3. Any patient with burns of more than 20 percent of the body.
4. Any patient with burns of 10 percent or more of the body and with heart, kidney, or liver disease or diabetes.
5. Any patient with signs of a respiratory problem.

BURN TREATMENT
Minor Burns
Burns of less than 10 percent of the body, unless deep, are usually treated on an ambulatory outpatient basis. Institute tetanus prophylaxis as outlined at the end of the chapter.

If only a small area is involved, cold water may be applied until the pain subsides.

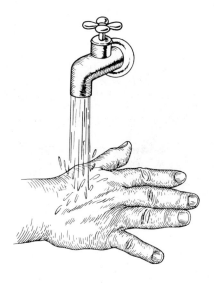

Debride all ruptured vesicles completely; do not open intact vesicles.

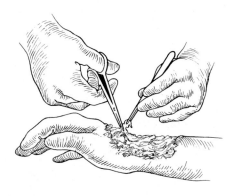

Apply fine-mesh gauze impregnated with a small amount of petroleum jelly or an antibiotic cream. Cover with three to four layers of coarse-mesh gauze and hold with a conforming gauze roller bandage. The dressing is usually changed in 3 to 4 days unless an odor is detected or the area becomes painful after 24 to 36 hours. Some superficial second-degree burns may be left exposed and washed three times daily with soap and water. A silver or other antibiotic cream is applied after each washing.

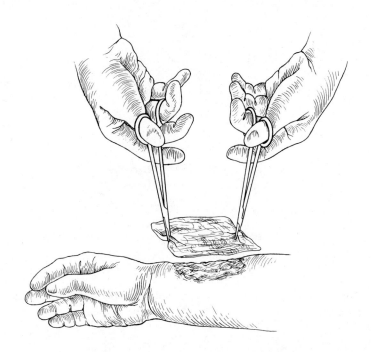

If infection is suspected, the wound should be cultured. Appropriate oral antibiotics should be reserved for patients with systemic symptoms. In larger burns, penicillin may be indicated to avoid streptococcal infection of the burn wound. At each dressing change, debride loose skin or necrotic material.

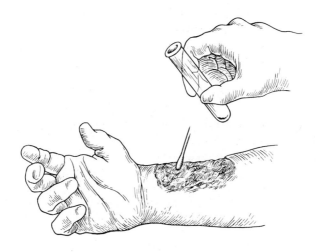

Burned hands and forearm must be splinted in the position of function.

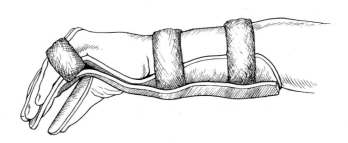

SUMMARY OF THE INITIAL TREATMENT OF SEVERE BURNS
1. Check to make sure that the patient's airway is open.
2. Cut down with a large-bore catheter into the cephalic vein in the shoulder area or the saphenous vein at the ankle. Start infusing Ringer's lactate.
3. Draw blood for typing, cross matching, blood urea nitrogen, a complete blood count, and electrolytes.
4. Institute tetanus prophylaxis.
5. Give intravenous morphine for pain; do not give intramuscular or subcutaneous medications for they may not be absorbed.
6. Insert a Foley catheter into the urinary bladder and monitor the output.
7. Wash the burned area gently with a mild soap and water and debride ruptured vesicles.
8. Cover the wound with a silver preparation or other antibacterial cream. Unless there is a history of allergy, penicillin is administered.

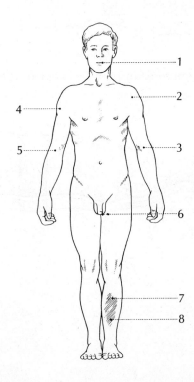

ESCHAROTOMY
Escharotomy is needed in circumferential burns of the trunk or of an extremity, since the burn eschar may restrict ventilation by preventing chest expansion, or the eschar may impair blood flow to an extremity. No anesthesia is required for the procedure, since the area of a third-degree burn is insensitive. The incision extends the full length of the burn eschar, through the full thickness of the skin, and into the subcutaneous tissue. Adequate release is indicated by separation of the eschar edges and improvement in ventilation, or circulation, or both.

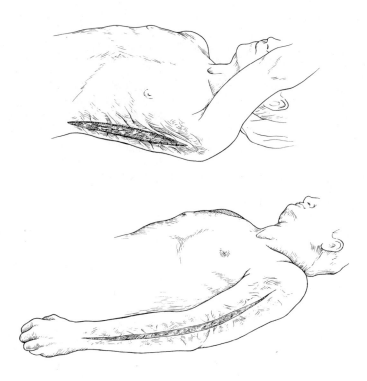

CHEMICAL BURNS
Chemical burns are not burns in the true sense, but rather are lesions produced by the interaction between the chemical and the body surface, external or internal. Treatment for various types of chemical burns is outlined in Table 15-1.

Table 15-1. Treatment of Chemical Burns

Oxidizing Agents
Examples: Chromic acid, chlorine disinfectants and bleaches, potassium permanganate
External treatment: Flush surface with water in copious amounts
Internal treatment: Milk, egg white, or aluminum hydroxide gels

Reducing Agents
Examples: Hydrochloric acid, nitric acid, alkyl mercury agents
External treatment: Debride all vesicles. Flush surface with soapy water
Internal treatment: Egg whites and/or aluminum hydroxide gels

Corrosives
Example: Phenol
External treatment: Flush with water and/or cover with oil
Internal treatment: Activated charcoal and demulcents

White Phosphorus
External treatment: Cover with water or oil to stop action, and excise the phosphorus-containing tissue
Internal treatment: Lavage with water or 1:5,000 dilution of potassium permanganate

Dichromate Salts
External treatment: Wash with water or 2% hyposulfite solution
Internal treatment: Lavage with water

Lyes
External treatment: Flush with water or weak acid solutions such as dilute vinegar. Then cover with olive oil
Internal treatment: Give nothing by mouth

Protoplasmic Poisons
Examples: Tungstic acid, picric acid, tannic acid, acetic acid, formic acid
External treatment: Flush with water
Internal treatment: Lavage with water

Metabolic Competitors
Examples: Hydrofluoric acid, oxalic acid
External treatment: If fluoride has penetrated the skin, local injection of calcium gluconate is indicated
Internal treatment: Gastric lavage with lime water (0.15% calcium hydroxide solution). May need IV calcium gluconate if signs of tetany develop

Desiccants
Examples: Sulfuric acid, muriatic acid (commercial grade hydrochloric acid)
External treatment: Do not only lavage with water. Flush area with lime water or wash with soap
Internal treatment: Lavage with lime water, then instill demulcents

Vesicants
Examples: Cantharides, dimethyl sulfoxide
External treatment: Wash with water
Internal treatment: Copious water lavage

Poison Gases
Examples: Mustard gas, lewisite
External treatment: Wash surface with oil or kerosene then soap and water
Internal treatment: Patient may need dimercaprol (BAL). Dosage is 2.5 mg per kilogram, administered at 4-hour intervals IM

GUIDE TO PROPHYLAXIS AGAINST TETANUS
IN WOUND MANAGEMENT*
Previously Immunized Persons
When the patient has been actively immunized within the past
10 years, the following rules apply:

1. To the great majority, give 0.5 ml of adsorbed tetanus toxoid
   as a booster unless it is certain that the patient has received a
   booster within the preceding 5 years.
2. To those with severe, neglected, or old (more than 24 hours)
   tetanus-prone wounds, give 0.5 ml of adsorbed tetanus toxoid
   unless it is certain that the patient has received a booster
   within the past year.

When the patient has been actively immunized more than 10
years previously the following rules apply:

1. To the great majority, give 0.5 ml of adsorbed tetanus toxoid.
2. To those with severe, neglected, or old (more than 24 hours)
   tetanus-prone wounds:

   a. Give 0.5 ml of adsorbed tetanus toxoid.
   b. Give 250 units of tetanus immune globulin (human).
   c. Consider administering oxytetracycline or penicillin.

Persons Not Previously Immunized
With clean minor wounds in which tetanus is most unlikely, give
0.5 ml of adsorbed tetanus toxoid (initial immunizing dose).

With all other wounds:

1. Give 0.5 ml of adsorbed tetanus toxoid (initial immunizing
   dose).
2. Give 250 units of tetanus immune globulin (human).
3. Consider administering oxytetracycline or penicillin.

*Adapted from the Committee on Trauma, American College of Surgeons.

The U.S. Public Health Service Advisory Committee on Immunization Practices in 1972 recommended diphtheria-pertussis-tetanus (DPT) vaccine for basic immunization in infants and children from 2 months through the sixth year and combined tetanus and diphtheria toxoids, adult type, to those over 6 years, unless sensitivity to the diphtheria toxoid is suspected.

When both tetanus toxoid and human immune globulin are administered, different syringes and different sites must be used.

If the wound is very severe or more than 24 hours old, 500 instead of 250 units of human immune globulin should be given.

When an initial dose of tetanus toxoid is administered, arrangements must be made to complete the immunizing series with a second 0.5 ml of toxoid at 6 weeks and 0.5 ml of toxoid at 6 months.

Index